CBD AND HEMP
REMEDIES

Also by Sandra Hinchliffe

Cannabis Spa at Home

High Tea

CBD Every Day

CBD AND HEMP
REMEDIES

A Quick & Easy Guide to Help You Destress, Relax, and Relieve Pain Using Cannabis Products

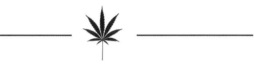

SANDRA HINCHLIFFE

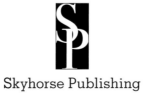

Skyhorse Publishing

Skyhorse Publishing books may be purchased in bulk at special discounts for sales promotion, corporate gifts, fund-raising, or educational purposes. Special editions can also be created to specifications. For details, contact the Special Sales Department, Skyhorse Publishing, 307 West 36th Street, 11th Floor, New York, NY 10018 or info@skyhorsepublishing.com.

Skyhorse® and Skyhorse Publishing® are registered trademarks of Skyhorse Publishing, Inc.®, a Delaware corporation.

Visit our website at www.skyhorsepublishing.com.

10 9 8 7 6 5 4 3 2 1

Library of Congress Cataloging-in-Publication Data is available on file.

Cover design by Daniel Brount
Cover photo credit: Sandra Hinchliffe

Print ISBN: 978-1-5107-5763-9
Ebook ISBN: 978-1-5107-5764-6

Printed in China

To all of the American hemp farmers, manufacturers, and retailers who have fought tirelessly to bring back hemp farming and production to our shores, creating a new base of manufacturing and jobs for our nation. Thank You.

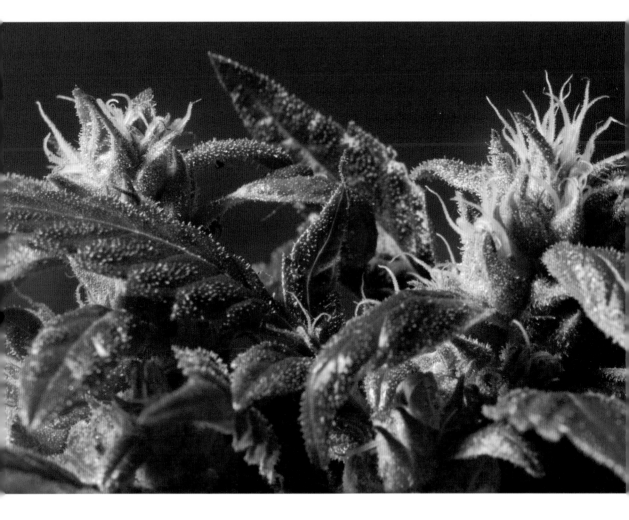

CONTENTS

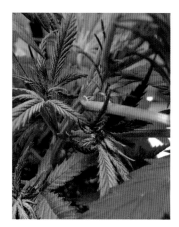

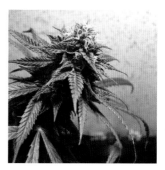

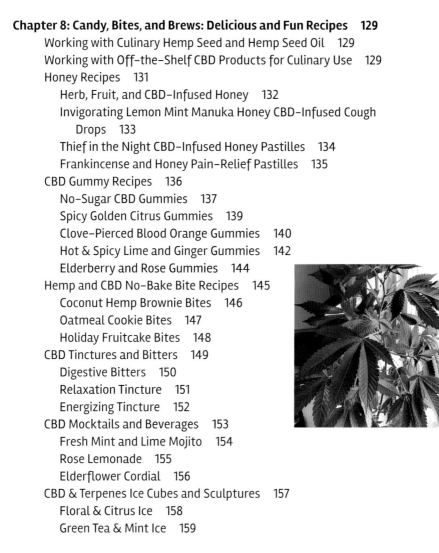

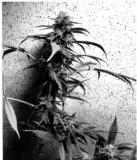

PREFACE

The home remedies, recipes, and techniques in this book are not intended as medical advice or treatment and are not a replacement for diagnosis and treatment from a licensed medical doctor.

Depending on your location, authentic CBD may or may not be legal. If you have questions regarding the legal use of CBD in your location, please consult an attorney.

The CBD recipes in this book are not intended for pregnant or nursing mothers or persons under the age of eighteen unless recommended and supervised by a licensed physician.

Culinary hemp seed and seed oil, and recipes that contain culinary hemp seed and seed oil, which do not contain cannabinoids (CBD, THC, etc.), are generally considered safe and nutritious for all ages, including pregnant or nursing mothers.

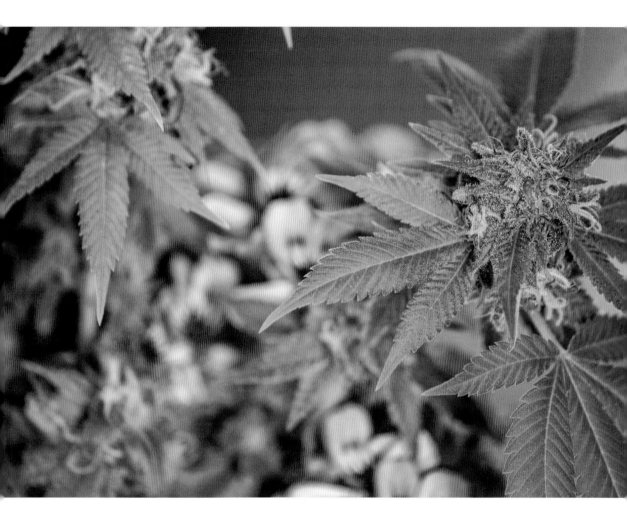

INTRODUCTION

Cannabis and Hemp are the Same Plant

Cannabis sativa L., a single species with three subspecies, *C. sativa subsp. sativa, C. sativa subsp. indica, C. sativa subsp. ruderalis,*[1,2] is one of the most fascinating plants in the world, with thousands of cultivars including what has been known as the drug cultivar of "marijuana" and the field crop known as hemp. *Marijuana* is not a botanical term, but rather a slang or popularized vernacular of Spanish-Mexican origin indicating that the cannabis plant or product that is being referenced is a drug variety. Any *Cannabis sativa L.* subspecies, and its cultivars, may have psychoactive properties due to higher THCA/THC content which may be referenced as "marijuana"—even official government institutions continue to use this slang or popular vernacular. Hemp, on the other hand references any *Cannabis sativa L.* subspecies cultivar that is selected for fiber and food production and for low THCA/THC content and/or higher CBDA/CBD content.

Marijuana, Cannabis, Hemp, Reefer, MaryJane, Indian Hemp, Ganja, The Devil's Cabbage—they're all the same plant. The classical medical text of the Middle Ages, Physica, authored by Hildegard von Bingen, both a saint and physician, describes hemp as a medicinal drug plant to be used topically and internally—and its psychoactive effects are noted in regard to a warning about its administration.[3]

---

1   Cannabis sativa, March 16, 2020 https://en.wikipedia.org/wiki/Cannabis_sativa
2   O'S News Service. *McPartland's Correct(ed) Vernacular Nomenclature*, January 4, 2015 https://beyondthc.com/mcpartlands-corrected-vernacular-nomenclature/
3   Von Bingen, Hildegard. *Physica*, translated from the Latin by Priscilla Throop. http://antiquecannabisbook.com/chap2B/West/WesternMedicine.htm

XI. HEMP "Hemp [hauff] is warm and grows where the air is neither very hot nor very cold, just as its nature is. Its seed is sound, and it is healthy for healthy people to eat it. It is openly gentle and useful in their stomach since it somewhat takes away the mucus. It is able to be digested easily; it diminishes the bad humors and makes the good humors strong. But nevertheless, whoever is weak in the head and has a vacant mind, if that person will have eaten hemp, it easily makes the person suffer pain somewhat in his or her head. However, whoever is sound in the head and has a full mind, it does not harm. Whoever is seriously ill, it also makes that person suffer pain somewhat in the stomach. However, whoever is only moderately ill, it does not cause pain when eaten.

"However, let whoever has a cold stomach cook hemp in water, squeeze out the water, wrap it in a cloth, and then place the hot cloth often over the stomach. This comforts the person and restores that place. Also, whoever has a vacant mind, if the person will have eaten hemp, it causes pain somewhat in the head; but it does not cause pain in a sound head and full brain. Also, the cloth made from the hemp heals ulcers and weeping wounds because the heat in the hemp has been tempered."

Under modern hemp regulation here in the United States, hemp is any cannabis plant producing any amount of CBD, but less than 0.3% THC.[4] And it is these cultivars that produce the CBD, hemp seed oil, hemp extracts, hemp foods, fiber, and home goods sold on retail shelves today. These

---

4   "Cannabis with a THC level exceeding 0.30 percent is considered marijuana, which remains classified as a schedule I controlled substance regulated by the Drug Enforcement Administration (DEA) under the CSA." *Establishment of a Domestic Hemp Production Program*, October 31, 2019. https://www.federalregister.gov/documents/2019/10/31/2019–23749/establishment -of-a-domestic-hemp-production-program

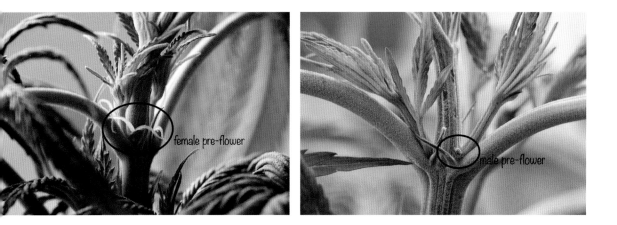

nonintoxicating cultivars of hemp contain varying amounts of CBDA/ CBD depending on many factors, such as genetics, growing environment, and growing technique like the selection of female to male plants.

Cannabis Anatomy 101

Cannabis sativa and subspecies are dioecious, that is, they have both female and male flowers that occur separately. Male plants typically grow faster and have thick and vigorous stems especially suited to fiber production. And while they contain less in the way of cannabinoid production of either CBD or THC, they do contain cannabinoids and can also be harvested for this purpose—although this is not particularly practical or desirable. Female cannabis plants, especially when males are removed from the crop, produce prolific flowers rich in cannabinoid and terpene content.

CBD and THC are the two cannabinoids that are best known. But there are actually more than a hundred cannabinoids that have been identified, along with dozens of terpenes, and these produce the variety

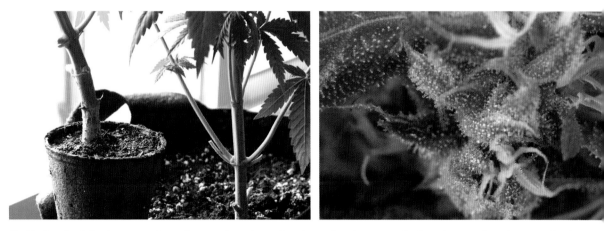

(Left) On the left, the stem of a male cannibas plant. On the right, the stem of a female cannabis plant. Both plants are the same age. Note the thicker stem of the male plant, which is well suited for commercial fiber production. (Right) Mature female cannabis flower with trichomes.

of fragrances found in the cultivars of *Cannabis sativa* and subspecies, including hemp.[5]

In most instances, the CBD and hemp products found at your favorite retail store are produced from a field crop of both male and female plants that meet the federal hemp regulatory standard of THC levels below 0.3%.

What Is CBD and How Is It Used?

CBD (cannabidiol) and CBDA (cannabidiolic acid), the acidic precursor to CBD, occur naturally in raw cannabis plant material in varying amounts. CBDA becomes CBD through the application of time (curing) and/or

5   UCLA Cannabis Research Initiative. "Cannabis and its Compounds." UCLAHealth.org. https://www.uclahealth.org/cannabis/cannabis-and-its-compounds

heat. Fresh cannabis will contain mostly CBDA, and this is heat-processed by the manufacturer of your favorite CBD oils and products to make the end product of CBD.

CBD/CBDA does not occur in any other plant species, including hops, tree bark, or orange peels. Consumers should not purchase products claiming unique methods for extracting CBD from any other plant other than cannabis. Unfortunately, there are many unscrupulous sellers entering the crowded CBD marketplace making claims that cannot be proven. Recently, as of the publication date of this book, there has been some legitimate research in regard to genetically engineered yeast designed to produce cannabinoids like CBD, but this technology is not available as a retail product for consumers or for wholesale at this time.[6]

CBD is both a retail herbal supplement product and an FDA-approved prescription-only medication.[7] It is one of the few compounds in the world to have this unique distinction. As of the publication of this book, this distinction, and more precisely, how the retail products should be classified, are an ongoing debate, as new legislation continues to be introduced in the United States and other countries.

If you have been prescribed Epidiolex, the prescription-only CBD medication, you will want to use that product precisely as instructed by your physician. Do not use this prescription-only CBD medication for recipes or home remedies. This prescription medication has only been approved by the FDA for certain types of epilepsy—but like other prescription medications, a licensed physician may prescribe it for off-label uses.

If you are purchasing CBD as a retail consumer product, you can use this product for recipes and home remedies that appeal to you. Both hemp products and CBD extractions can be used as culinary, spa, home remedy,

---

6   "Yeast produce low-cost, high-quality cannabinoids." University of California–Berkeley. February 27, 2019. https://www.sciencedaily.com/releases/2019/02/190227131838.htm

7   Epidiolex, GW Pharmaceuticals. https://www.epidiolex.com/

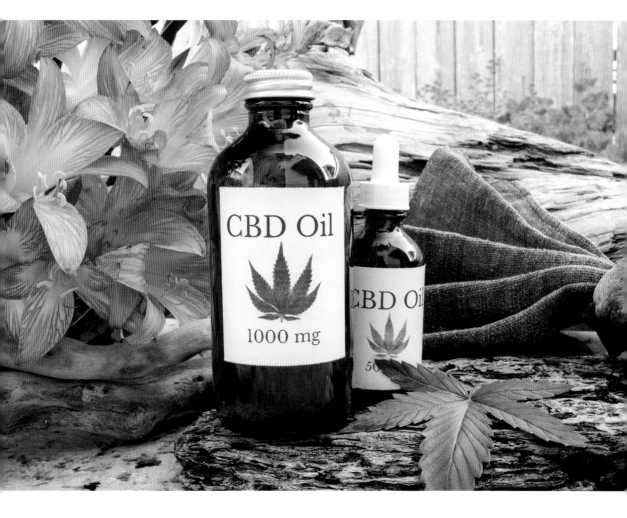

or sober recreational products. Hemp products, such as culinary hemp seed oil, hemp seed, and hemp fiber clothing, are safe for most people and appropriate for all ages, CBD products, like some other supplements and beauty products sold in the retail marketplace, are not for everyone. And as with some other supplements and beauty products, consumers should be aware that overuse or misuse could lead to unwanted side effects. For example, retail CBD supplement products are not appropriate for treating or curing diseases or medical conditions. Also, as you would with any supplement product, consult your physician if you have questions about using it with prescribed medications or if you have questions about appropriate dosages.

Typically, the labeling on CBD products will suggest dosages and serving sizes, and these are a good place to start when trying CBD for the first time. Many beginners will want to start with very small doses—this method, known as microdosing, ranges from 0.25 to 3 milligrams of CBD per serving.

What About Hemp Seed and Hemp Seed Oil?

Hemp seed and hemp seed oil are produced from crops of field hemp. The female plants of these crops produce the seed, which is cold-pressed for the oil or harvested for the seed alone.

Hemp seed and hemp seed oil are used in countless products: wellness supplements, culinary products, and spa products. They are also sold as stand-alone products in many retail stores. Both hemp seed and hemp seed oil are free of THC and CBD. Serving sizes of these two products will be indicated on labels, and these products are safe for consumption by people of all ages.

Are Hemp and CBD Legal?

Although hemp is legal on the federal level in the United States, as it is in many other countries, your local government may consider CBD either legal or illegal. Culinary hemp seed oil, hemp seed, and hemp fiber (finished products such as clothing and paper) are legal and available in every state and many countries in the world and have been available as a stand-alone retail and wholesale product for many more years than CBD! Prior to the modern legalization of hemp farming in the United States, these products were imported from, and continue to be imported from, Canada and Europe, where hemp farming has always been legal.

Most large retail chains carry a variety of hemp products in 2020. You'll find hemp seed oil and shelled seed, as well as lotions and balms and other finished products, such as clothing and linens. And in locations where retail CBD products are legal, you'll find CBD oils, concentrates, and finished, CBD-infused products on the shelves of many major retail stores.

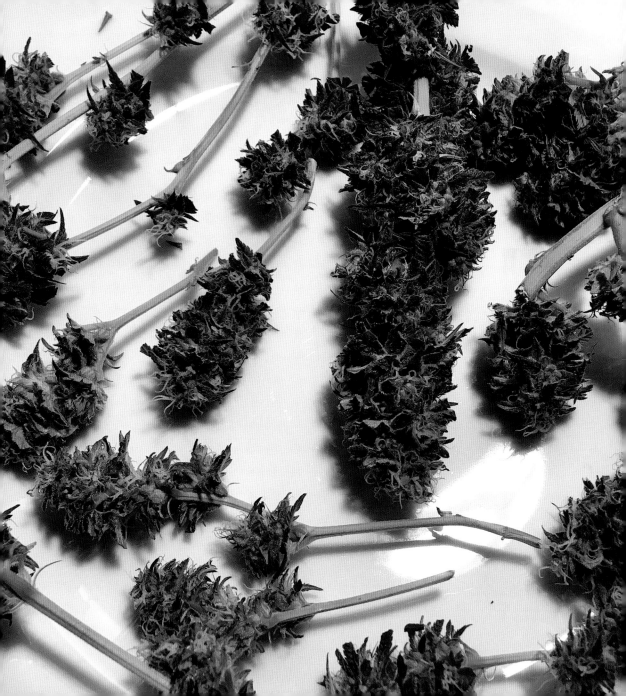

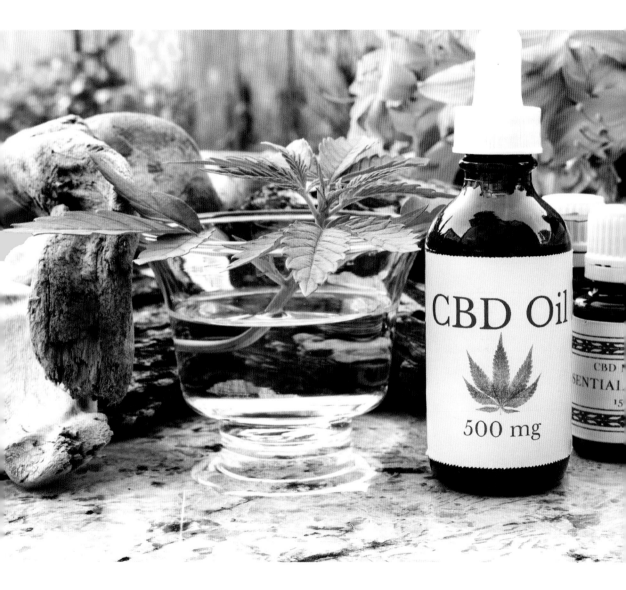

CHAPTER ONE

HEMP AND CBD: PRODUCTS AND SELECTION

A new legal framework for cannabis in the United States and other countries, beginning in the twenty-first century, has created a new retail product industry. In this chapter, we will learn about the wide variety of hemp and CBD products available to consumers and how to select and use these products.

Hemp Products: What You Need to Know

Consumers will obtain the best results and the most satisfaction by purchasing hemp products from companies with transparency, ethical branding, and clear labeling.

The Cannabis sativa subspecies, which comprise the hemp cultivar products available to consumers, are powerful remediators of the soil and absorb environmental toxins and heavy metals present in the soil. For this reason, purchasing products from companies with a commitment to farmers (who care about the health of the soil or other growing medium that their hemp is grown in) is the best way to begin to evaluate the quality of any hemp or CBD product that you want to purchase.

Products from companies who disclose the origins of their hemp and third-party test results for CBD or hemp extracts will be the products of the highest quality—irrespective of price.

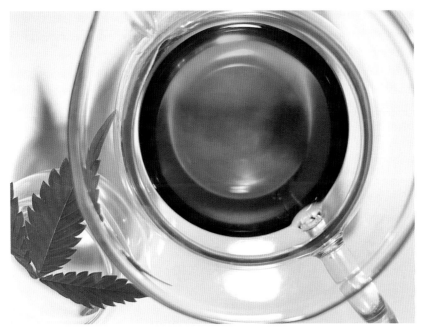

Hemp Seed Oil

Hemp seed oil is the cold-pressed oil from the seeds of field hemp female flowers. It is high in omega and polyunsaturated fatty acids, which makes it a nourishing oil for culinary purposes as well as skin care products and spa applications, such as massage oil.

There are two types of hemp seed oil:

1. **Cold-pressed raw and unrefined.** Light to darker green in color, this oil contains some of the natural fragrance of hemp due to its unrefined state but does not have any cannabinoid content, such as CBD or THC. This oil is available for purchase at many major retail and big-box stores.

When purchasing this product, it is best to purchase it from retailers who store the oil in refrigerated cases. Purchase and use this oil before the expiration date printed on the bottle. Don't purchase unrefined hemp seed oil that does not have an expiration date printed on the bottle.

This form of hemp seed oil is the preferred form for culinary applications and is very heat- and environmentally sensitive. Unrefined hemp seed oil should never be heated for cooking applications, such as frying or baking, and should be kept in a dark container and a cool environment. Typically, the best place to store fresh, unrefined hemp seed oil is in a dark container and in the refrigerator until it is ready for use in recipes.

Unrefined hemp seed oil is a very delicate oil and requires special handling when used in culinary applications and for skin care or spa due to the possibility of rancidity. A rancid oil will smell "off" or stale and not have the fresh "grassy" fragrance of stable oil. The flavor of unrefined hemp seed oil should be light, nutty, and slightly grassy with no unpleasant fragrances or flavors.

Unrefined hemp seed oil, when used for skin, hair, or in spa applications, has a shorter shelf life than many other oils. It is suggested to pair with antioxidants, such as rosemary antioxidant, to protect the oil from rancidity to extend the shelf life. In the spa and topical recipes that contain hemp seed oil that follow this chapter, rosemary antioxidant is the preferred antioxidant.

Treat unrefined hemp seed oil the way that you would treat any fine culinary luxury or precious herb—with great care that will extend the life of the oil.

2. **Cold-pressed refined oil.** This oil will have a clear or very light color and is neutral to lightly fragrant. It does not contain any cannabinoids, such as CBD or THC. Because it is refined, it has a longer shelf

life than unrefined oil if kept in the same optimal conditions as you would keep the unrefined oil. It should be noted that refined hemp seed oil is not used in culinary applications. Refined hemp seed oil is not typically sold in retail or big-box stores but can be purchased online from shops specializing in manufacturing oils for the cosmetic or craft industry.

Typically, refined oil is used in mass consumer products, such as lotion and soap, due to the extended shelf life, whereas unrefined oil will be found in more artisan products. Refined hemp seed oil has many of the same properties as the unrefined oil, including being one of the few oils for skin and hair with the lowest comedogenic ratings.[8] Use refined hemp seed oil within one to two years from the date of purchase for best results in any application. It is also recommended that refined hemp seed oil is paired with an antioxidant, such as rosemary, to prevent rancidity in most finished spa and topical products.

Refined hemp seed oil also has many uses beyond skin care, hair care, and spa—including paint, varnish, biofuel, and bioplastics production. It also makes a wonderful eco-friendly wood polish—try this recipe at home to revive wood surfaces on furniture and decor like wood frames: Combine 3 drops of lemon essential oil and ¼ cup (60ml) hemp seed oil in a glass bottle. Shake thoroughly and apply to a soft cloth and use on wood surfaces as needed.

Shelled Hemp Seed

Shelled hemp seed is the raw, oily "nut" of the hemp seed produced by female field hemp plants. It has a nutty flavor and can be used in many of the same culinary applications as tree nuts and seeds. Like hemp seed oil, it does not contain any cannabinoids, such as CBD or THC.

---

8   "Comedogenic Ratings (Causes Acne)." SkinReference.com. http://www.skinreference.com .php72-6.phx1-2.websitetestlink.com/comedogenic-ratings-causes-acne/

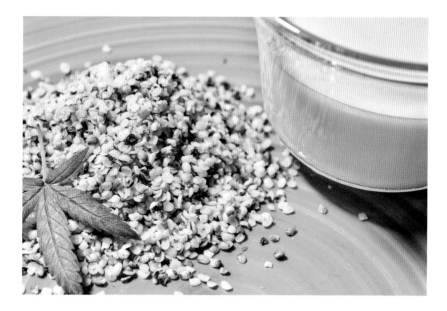

Hemp seed is not a nut but is classified as a seed and does not have the same allergenic proteins as tree nuts or peanuts, which makes it safe for consumption by those with tree nut and peanut allergies as long as it is shelled and produced in factories free of tree nut and peanut production.

Shelled hemp seed is a raw product that can go rancid quite easily when exposed to heat, light, and oxygen for extended periods of time. It should be stored in refrigeration in a dark and tightly closed container and used by the expiration date printed on the package. Shelled hemp seed is a popular product and available at many grocery stores. It is best to purchase this product when the retailer stores it in refrigeration or on a cool shelf in the store.

Shelled hemp seed is high in both complete proteins and omega fatty acids. It's a great addition to smoothies, salads, and desserts as a crust or topping. It also makes a delightful "milk" or "cream" that can be used in similar ways as dairy or nut milks, sans cooking. Shelled hemp seed can withstand a moderate amount of heat, such as inclusion in a topping for muffins or cake, or in crusts, but should not be exposed to heat for extended periods of time.

Make a simple hemp nut milk in your blender that is delicious and creamy: ⅓ cup (80 g) of shelled hemp seed, 1 cup (240 ml) of cold water, and a few small cubes of ice. You may add a little vanilla extract for enhanced flavor if you desire. Process in the blender until smooth and milky. Drink immediately for best flavor, but it can be stored for up to 1 day in the refrigerator.

Hemp Protein

Hemp protein is extracted from shelled hemp seed and concentrated to create a protein-rich powder that can be used in smoothies, shakes, and many other recipes just like other kinds of protein powders. Like shelled hemp seed, it is sensitive to environmental exposure and heat. Hemp protein should be kept in a tightly sealed container and in the refrigerator after opening. Use this product by its expiration date for the best taste and results. Hemp protein, depending on the brand, generally has more of an "herbal" flavor than other protein powders like pea or even whey protein—keep this in mind when using it in your recipes. Hemp protein does not contain THC or CBD.

Whole Hemp Seed

Whole hemp seed, in contrast to shelled hemp seed, has not had its hard seed coat removed. This makes whole hemp seed more shelf-stable than shelled hemp seed—but this product is best when refrigerated and should be used before the expiration date printed on the package. Like shelled hemp seed, it can withstand moderate heat in culinary applications, such as toppings or crusts.

Whole hemp seed is typically toasted by the manufacturer before it is packaged for sale. This improves the flavor and crunch and renders the seed

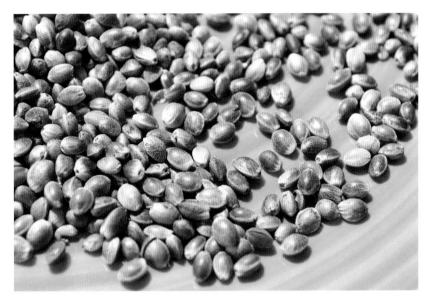

sterile. Whole hemp seed is appropriate for baked goods and any culinary application where extra crunch and fiber are desired and does not contain CBD or THC.

This product can be found in natural foods or specialty grocers and is less common than shelled hemp seed.

Hemp Fiber Goods

Hemp fiber is the bast fiber of the hemp stalk, which is used to make a variety of consumer goods like fabrics and paper. Field hemp is a fast-growing crop that can replace both wood and cotton in many products. Hemp hurds and fiber are used in many novel applications, such as home insulation, bricks, plastics, rope, and twine. Hemp fibers have long lives and are not as prone to rot as other kinds of fibers.

Because hemp is a fast-growing crop, more products can be produced from a field of hemp than from the same area planted with trees or

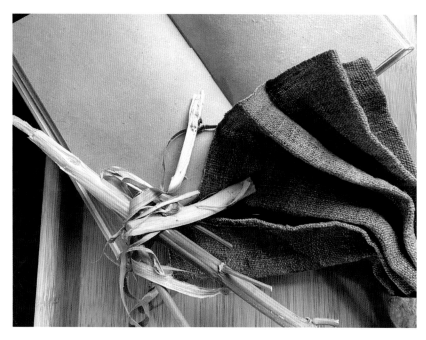

cotton—and hemp does not require the chemicals used to farm cotton and other fiber crops. Hemp is ideal for clothing due to the long life of the fiber and is very environmentally friendly. Hemp fiber goods do not contain THC or CBD and are safe for all ages.

Hemp Extracts

Hemp extracts can vary depending on how a maker or manufacturer defines this product. Typically, an *herbal extract* or *tincture* is going to be a whole plant infused into a solvent like alcohol. The final product can be a liquid tincture or resinous oil with all of the constituents of the hemp plant, including cannabinoids and terpenes. Hemp extracts may not be completely free of THC, and, for that reason, these products are not recommended for those who do not want any THC or a trace of THC in

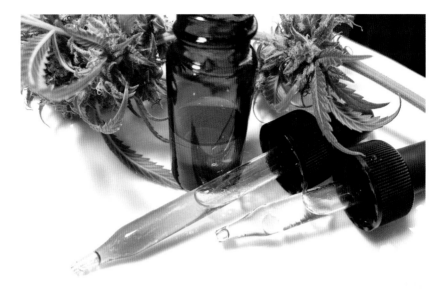

the hemp products they consume. They are, however, legal to sell in many places if they meet the federal regulatory standard of 0.3% THC or less.

Some products labeled as "hemp extract" may only be hemp seed oil and not a "true" extract or tincture. Hemp seed oil contains only oil pressed from the seeds of the hemp plant and nothing else. These products should be labeled as "hemp seed oil," but unfortunately, some unscrupulous sellers and manufacturers will call this an extract and sell it for prices that far exceed what one would pay for properly labeled hemp seed oil from their local grocery store. Hemp extracts may or may not be labeled with cannabinoid content—but a responsible manufacturer will provide third-party test results that verify the cannabinoid content to consumers for products labeled as "hemp extract."

Hemp extracts should be stored away from light or heat and used by the expiration date printed on the bottle or jar.

CBD: Full-Spectrum or Isolate?

CBD products come in two types: full-spectrum and isolate. **Full-spectrum** is a whole-plant product and can be extracted from any aerial part of the hemp plant. This CBD product will have chlorophyll and other constituents of the hemp plant, including terpenes and a full spectrum of cannabinoids, with CBD as the primary cannabinoid. Full-spectrum products, while meeting the US federal regulations for THC content, may not be suitable for consumers who wish to avoid THC.

CBD isolate is a unique product in that it is the isolated CBD molecule—and this can be a versatile cannabinoid for manufacturing CBD products completely free of THC content. Most of the CBD products on the shelves of major retail stores in 2020 are products manufactured with the isolated CBD molecule.

In the recipe chapters of this book, you will find many suggestions for getting the most out of either full-spectrum or isolated CBD. Your selection of one or both of these products will depend on location and retail availability in your area, or legalities of shipment to your area.

CBD Oil and Concentrates

CBD oil can be either full-spectrum or isolated CBD. CBD oil is CBD in a carrier oil such as olive, coconut (MCT), or any other oil or butter. CBD oil can also be concentrated as a resinous oil by reducing it from an alcohol-based tincture, or through other methods such as CO2 extraction and isolated separations of cannabinoids such as CBDA/CBD. These methods of extraction can create full-spectrum oils and resins as well as CBD isolates that are at least 99% pure.

These products can be used neat, or in recipes with herbal and aroma entourage to potentiate or complement their benefits. CBD oil may have THC content below federal regulations, or no THC content at all.

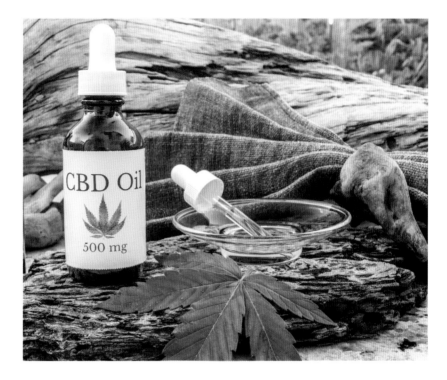

Full-spectrum oils almost always have THC content below the federally regulated amount, while isolated CBD oil will be THC-free.

Water-Soluble CBD

CBD and CBDA are resinous molecules that require suspension in oil carriers or emulsifiers for even distribution in water-based products, such as water-soluble CBD products. Water-soluble CBD can be used neat or in many different recipes that have water as an ingredient, such as bath preparations. Edible water-soluble CBD products can be used in tea or other water-based beverages. Emulsifiers for CBD include gels, gums, and surfactants.

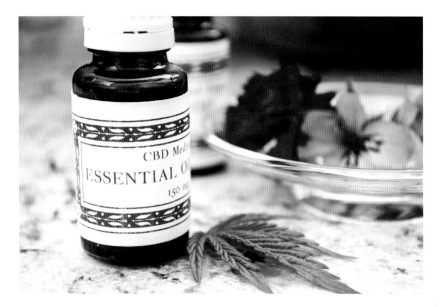

CBD Infusions

CBD infusions comprise another class of products, such as essential oils and blends that can be added to recipes, added to a diffuser, or used in CBD aromatherapy applications, for example. Some infusion products are also water soluble, such as water infused with CBD. These products should also have a manufacturing date or expiration date, or both, printed on the box, bottle, or jar, along with accessible test results.

Most recently, some manufacturers have been offering dry goods to consumers that are CBD-infused, such as pillows, pillowcases, and even mattresses. It is up to the consumer to decide if these products are useful for them—but the caveat is that most of these products will not come with test results.

Manufactured Hemp and CBD-infused Products

Finished products containing both hemp and CBD infusions are a convenient way for consumers to enjoy both hemp and CBD. It is the recommendation of the author of this book to purchase products that follow the good farming and manufacturing standards explained earlier in this chapter.

All finished products—including oils, lotions, beverages, candies, snacks, and more—should have a date of manufacture or expiration, or ideally both. Fresh products are important, as cannabinoids like CBD degrade with time. Hemp products, such as baked goods with hemp seed and hemp seed milk, have shorter shelf lives, and products that incorporate hemp ingredients are best used when fresh.

Cannabis Flower Essences

Methods of Flower Essence Production

The classical method of flower essence production was popularized by Edward Bach. His was a method of intuitive experience, with live flowers in the wild or in the garden that were then floated in spring water in sunlight for several hours, strained, and bottled with an equal amount of brandy. This formed the basis of what is known as *the mother tincture*. From the mother tincture, successive tinctures could be made using only a drop or two diluted in spring water and equal parts of brandy, and further dilutions could be obtained from that, with each succession always the same formulation of equal parts of water and brandy.

Cannabis Flower Essence Production and Selection

Cannabis flower essence follows a similar method—depending on the herbal artisan making and bottling it, it will contain varying subjective vibrational properties. Select a product you feel the greatest energetic connection with from a maker committed to the crafting of flower essences in an authentic manner. Keep these cannabis flower essence products stored in the manner suggested by the maker.

You can even make your own cannabis flower essences if you're in a location where living, fresh cannabis or hemp flowers are available to you! If the latter is intriguing to you, or you would like to learn more about a method of artisan cannabis flower essence production that you can do at home or for a professional spa, you will find instructions in chapter 5, section Cannabis Flower Essence Complementary (page 56).

Test Results: Why Companies Should Provide These and How to Read and Verify Test Results

Third-party test results made available to consumers by companies who manufacture CBD products indicate an ethical and quality standard that is consumer-centric. These should be provided on the labeling of products, such as a QR code, or in an easily accessible area of a manufacturer's website or app.

Reading these test results should not be difficult for the consumer:

1. The test results should contain levels of all cannabinoids in the product, including, but not limited to, CBD or CBDA.
2. The test results should contain information about the levels of microbial contamination or soil toxicity, such as heavy metal content. Testing for other toxicity, such as adulterated chemicals, should be detailed in the test results.
3. The best-quality test results will also contain information about the presence of terpenes, including testing for any artificially produced terpene content.

To verify third-party test results, look on the document that has been generated by the testing facility and do a search for this facility online. A reputable manufacturer will not have affiliation with or ownership of their own testing facility. Testing facilities should also have proper licensing, which will be regulated at the state level and can be verified by visiting the state agency that regulates licenses for these facilities. Finally, contact with the facility listed on the test results document can confirm the authenticity of the test performed by that facility.

Product Selection and Tasting Notes

In this section, you can test and evaluate the products you have tried at home! As a beginner, you'll want to create a selection and tasting journal that acts as a unique guide to the products you have enjoyed the most.

Date of Purchase	Place of Purchase	Product Name	Price	CBD Test Results? Y/N
Use and Tasting Notes				

Date of Purchase	Place of Purchase	Product Name	Price	CBD Test Results? Y/N

Use and Tasting Notes

Date of Purchase	Place of Purchase	Product Name	Price	CBD Test Results? Y/N

Use and Tasting Notes

Date of Purchase	Place of Purchase	Product Name	Price	CBD Test Results? Y/N

Use and Tasting Notes

Date of Purchase	Place of Purchase	Product Name	Price	CBD Test Results? Y/N

Use and Tasting Notes

Date of Purchase	Place of Purchase	Product Name	Price	CBD Test Results? Y/N

Use and Tasting Notes

Date of Purchase	Place of Purchase	Product Name	Price	CBD Test Results? Y/N

Use and Tasting Notes

Date of Purchase	Place of Purchase	Product Name	Price	CBD Test Results? Y/N

Use and Tasting Notes

Date of Purchase	Place of Purchase	Product Name	Price	CBD Test Results? Y/N

Use and Tasting Notes

Date of Purchase	Place of Purchase	Product Name	Price	CBD Test Results? Y/N

Use and Tasting Notes

Date of Purchase	Place of Purchase	Product Name	Price	CBD Test Results? Y/N

Use and Tasting Notes

Date of Purchase	Place of Purchase	Product Name	Price	CBD Test Results? Y/N

Use and Tasting Notes

Date of Purchase	Place of Purchase	Product Name	Price	CBD Test Results? Y/N

Use and Tasting Notes

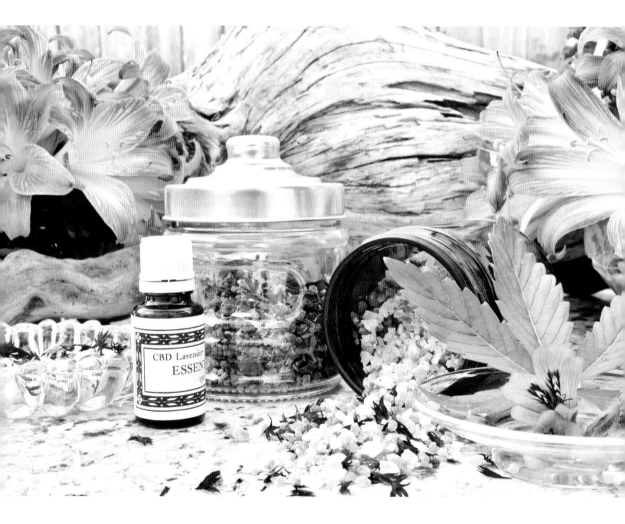

CHAPTER TWO

THE FOUNDATION OF RECIPE TECHNIQUE: HEMP, CBD, TERPENES, AND TOOLS

Get the most out of your favorite hemp and CBD products by learning terpene pairing. In this chapter, we will learn about the entourage effect, terpenes, and how to build an essential oil and herbal seasoning kit to enhance every experience with hemp and CBD.

Terpenes: What Are They and What Do They Do?

Sesquiterpenes and monoterpenes, collectively referred to as *terpenes*, as well as other types of fragrant volatile compounds, are the molecular building blocks of the fragrances we find in hemp and all varieties of cannabis. The same terpenes in cannabis can be found in many other aromatic plants, as nature has a habit of repeating what works! In this chapter, our primary focus will be on terpenes—with a few other fragrant compounds explored as points of interest. Terpenes are most easily understood as the language and defense system of plants. These fragrant compounds are released by plants to signal to the outside world an invitation to visit or pollinate a plant—as well as a defense to serve as an insecticide, fungicide, or antibacterial.

For humans, these natural fragrances are attractive, with many perceived benefits. You may already be familiar with them in the form of bottled essential oils, which are a collection of terpenes from an aromatic plant in the form of concentrated volatile oil. Terpenes contribute to what is known as the "entourage effect" of cannabis. This effect has been noted by many researchers and medical professionals, such as Dr. Sanjay Gupta, who was the first to discuss it with a wider, mainstream audience on his popular *Weed* series on CNN. All forms of cannabis and cannabinoids, including CBD, are more effective with an entourage that includes these delightful natural fragrances.

Regardless of the kind of CBD oil, CBD concentrate, hemp extract, or other hemp product you would like to work with to deliver your CBD or hemp aromatherapy experience, you can create the entourage effect using essential oils and many of the basic kitchen herbs and spices you are already familiar with.

Cannabis Terpenes Found in Other Plants

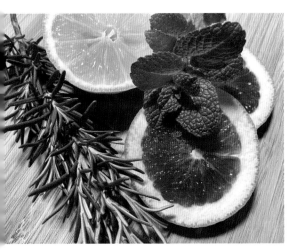

This chart will help you identify some of the terpenes in cannabis found in other plants that will create the desired effects and benefits in the aromatherapy recipes and techniques in the following chapters. This chart represents a few of the most common terpenes found in cannabis and a few examples of their corresponding essential oils.

Terpene Chart for Pairing with CBD and Hemp

Terpene	Essential Oil	Therapeutic Effects
Pinene	pine, rosemary	motivating, enlivening
Linalool	lavender, sweet basil	relieving, calming
Limonene	lemon, orange (citrus)	energizing, brightening
Geraniol	rose, rose geranium	cooling, uplifting
Myrcene	lemongrass, thyme	potentiating, relaxing
Caryophyllene	black pepper, cloves, carnation	anti-inflammatory, anxiolytic
Humulene	hops, cannabis	digestif, soothing
Cineole	eucalyptus, tea tree	invigorating, refreshing

Essential Oils

The easiest way to identify a specific terpene in any essential oil is to look for the certificate of analysis for the specific oil you would like to purchase. All reputable essential oil companies post their COA (certificate of analysis) on their websites or make their third-party testing certificates available to consumers. These certificates contain a wealth of information about the specific levels of each terpene in every batch of essential oil. Since many essential oils can have variations in their terpene content from batch to batch, reviewing the COA is the most reliable way to determine if an essential oil contains the desired terpene content to pair with your favorite CBD, hemp extract, or hemp oil product for an aromatherapeutic experience or recipe.

The other advantage of including this step when selecting essential oils as an entourage for CBD or hemp is that it will enable you to eliminate

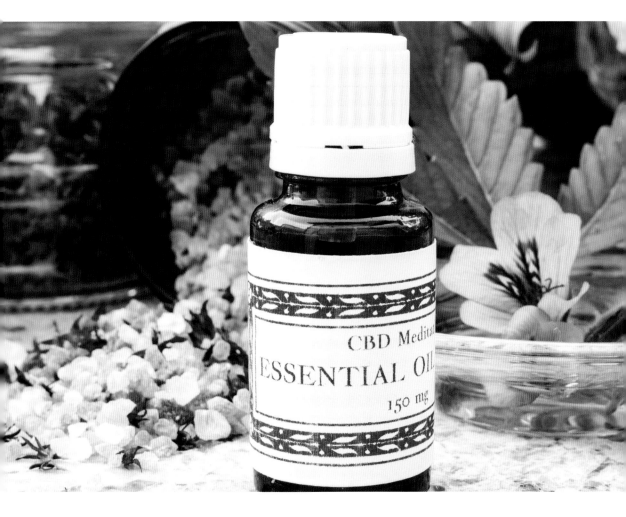

essential oils that have been adulterated with artificial ingredients, as this is unfortunately more common than many consumers realize.

Working with Essential Oils, CBD, and Hemp

In this chapter, you are learning about essential oils, the aromatic plants that produce terpenes, and how these correspond and pair with the naturally occurring aromatic terpenes in cannabis. In the chapters that follow, you will learn about specific aromatherapeutic recipes and spa techniques to which you can apply your newly acquired knowledge about pairing terpenes with CBD and hemp to get the most benefits and enjoyment from them.

Essential Oil Best Practices

Let's look at some of the caveats of working with essential oils. The first principle in working with essential oils for any purpose is *less is more*. Just because essential oils are the terpene product of plants doesn't mean that these oils can be used in copious amounts in everything without consequences that could endanger your health.

Essential oils are a serious herbal preparation requiring mindfulness. For a moment, let's put aside potential health issues, such as sensitization and chemical burns, and discuss one other aspect of overuse and misuse that may occur when eating essential oils, using them undiluted or under-diluted, or using them for extended periods of time—olfactory fatigue or nose blindness. Via the overuse and misuse of essential oils, one can cease to obtain any of the benefits by experiencing the loss of the ability to detect the subtle nuances of every terpene you encounter. To get the most out of your hemp or CBD experience, you will want to use essential oils judiciously—always dilute and never consume orally.

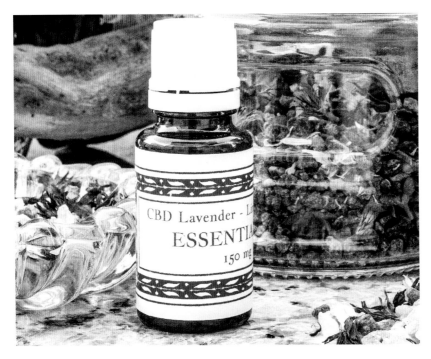

Phototoxicity

Some essential oils are known to potentiate the effects of sun exposure—this is known as *phototoxicity*. You will want to avoid applying any phototoxic essential oil, even diluted, to the skin and then exposing yourself to the sun for at least twelve hours after application. The addition of CBD or hemp oil will not ameliorate this effect.

Some of the most common phototoxic essential oils are: all citrus such as orange, lemon, grapefruit, and bergamot; cumin; rue; and angelica. Some citrus essential oils are considered lower risk when steam-distilled instead of cold-pressed. If you aren't sure of the phototoxicity of an essential oil, treat it as you would a phototoxic essential oil and do not expose yourself to the sun after application to the skin.

Sensitization

Some essential oils are known to have a greater potential for sensitization in individuals with immune systems prone to sensitization. This can range from rashes and hives to more serious and life-threatening allergic reactions, such as anaphylactic shock. Once an individual is sensitized to an essential oil, they can never use it again without severe risk.

The most common essential oils responsible for sensitization are: peppermint, lavender, lemongrass, and cinnamon. Judicious use and dilution of these essential oils when pairing with CBD and hemp will help prevent sensitization.

Furthermore, some essential oils are not appropriate for pregnant women, babies, children, and pets. Because these are so varied, before you use any essential oil around or on pregnant women, babies, children, and pets, it's suggested you consult your licensed physician or veterinarian first—even if you plan to only use them with hemp products (hemp seed oil, hemp soap, etc.) that do not contain CBD or any other cannabinoid and are generally considered safe for pregnant women, babies, children, and pets as singular products.

Essential Oil Kit Planner

Included in this section are suggestions for planning and assembling an essential oil kit to complement your favorite CBD or hemp product. Some suggestions for your first essential oil kit representing the most common terpenes in cannabis are: sweet orange, lemon, clove, eucalyptus, rosemary, pine, lavender, geranium, lemongrass, frankincense, and black pepper. With these, you will be able to create a variety of aromas to enhance any CBD or hemp recipe or spa experience. As you begin to develop your own CBD and hemp aromatherapeutics, you can add more essential oils to your repertoire. Get started with your own experimentation with essential oil terpenes by using this essential oil kit planner for pairing with CBD and hemp.

1. Record the kind of essential oil, brand, and price. Check the COA from the manufacturer to determine the terpene content and write down the primary terpene content from the COA. These will be listed in order of concentration on the report. Essential oils will have a combination of terpenes, but there will always be one or two terpenes that are the most concentrated in the oil, and these are the ones you will record as the primary terpenes.
2. What will you blend or pair with this essential oil? If you will be creating a blend or pairing with another essential oil for use with your favorite CBD or hemp product, write that down so that you remember this recipe and the proportions of oil you use.
3. Test blend experiments in a water-based diffuser for best results when composing recipe blends.
4. Record your fragrance notes and any recipe experimentation with other essential oils—don't forget to note if any of these have potential photosensitivity so that you can plan for appropriate use during sun exposure. Note your aromatherapy experience and any therapeutic effects such as calming, pain relief, etc.

Essential Oil	Brand	Price	Primary Terpenes	Blends and Pairings

Fragrance and Experience Notes

Essential Oil	Brand	Price	Primary Terpenes	Blends and Pairings

Fragrance and Experience Notes

Essential Oil	Brand	Price	Primary Terpenes	Blends and Pairings

Fragrance and Experience Notes

Essential Oil	Brand	Price	Primary Terpenes	Blends and Pairings

Fragrance and Experience Notes

Essential Oil	Brand	Price	Primary Terpenes	Blends and Pairings

Fragrance and Experience Notes

Essential Oil	Brand	Price	Primary Terpenes	Blends and Pairings

Fragrance and Experience Notes

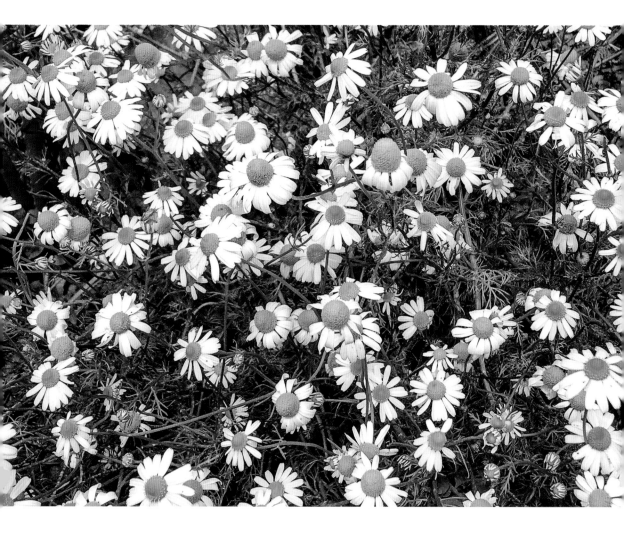

Pairing Aromatic Plants with CBD and Hemp

Whole aromatic plants have a few advantages over essential oils—the first being that, in many instances, the pairing you create with whole aromatics and CBD or hemp will be edible. Whole aromatic plants are much less concentrated in volatile oil and terpenes than essential oils. Additionally, whole aromatic plants are more budget-friendly than the exact same aromatherapy experience you can get with essential oils. Whole aromatics are also more nuanced and have more of a fresh fragrance than bottled essential oils, which makes them a great choice for pairing as terpene entourage with your favorite CBD or hemp products.

Spices and Whole Aromatic Plants Terpene Chart

Similar to the previous chart of essential oils and their corresponding terpenes in the cannabis plant, this chart represents some of the most common terpenes found in cannabis, as well as examples of spices and other whole aromatics that also produce these terpenes along with their purported therapeutic effects. You may find that quite a few of these are already in your kitchen spice rack—and that is the best place to start your adventure when pairing whole aromatics with your favorite CBD or hemp product!

Terpene	Edible Whole Aromatic	Therapeutic Effects
Pinene	sage, rosemary, frankincense resin	motivating, enlivening
Linalool	lavender, sweet basil	relieving, calming
Limonene	citrus peels	energizing, brightening
Geraniol	rose, rose geranium	cooling, uplifting
Myrcene	lemongrass, mango, thyme	potentiating, relaxing
Caryophyllene	black pepper, cloves, Ceylon cinnamon	anti-inflammatory, anxiolytic
Carvone	spearmint, wild mint, caraway seed	digestif, soothing

Working with Spices and Whole Aromatic Plants—Spices and Aromatics Kit Planner

Whole aromatic spices and herbs, whether purchased from a retail store or grown in your own garden, do not come with a COA like reputable essential brands do. There are two fundamental rules for getting the most out of whole aromatics: 1) look for retail products that are very fresh and 2) look for those that are preferably certified organic. The chart included here is brief—but any herb or spice can be researched online in order to determine their primary terpene content. Start with the chart here and then use the planner to formulate your own spice and herbal blends to pair with CBD and hemp along with the recipes you wish to develop.

Herb or Spice	Primary Terpenes	Blends and Pairings
Fragrance and Experience Notes		

Herb or Spice	Primary Terpenes	Blends and Pairings

Fragrance and Experience Notes

Herb or Spice	Primary Terpenes	Blends and Pairings

Fragrance and Experience Notes

Herb or Spice	Primary Terpenes	Blends and Pairings

Fragrance and Experience Notes

Herb or Spice	Primary Terpenes	Blends and Pairings

Fragrance and Experience Notes

Herb or Spice	Primary Terpenes	Blends and Pairings

Fragrance and Experience Notes

Herb or Spice	Primary Terpenes	Blends and Pairings

Fragrance and Experience Notes

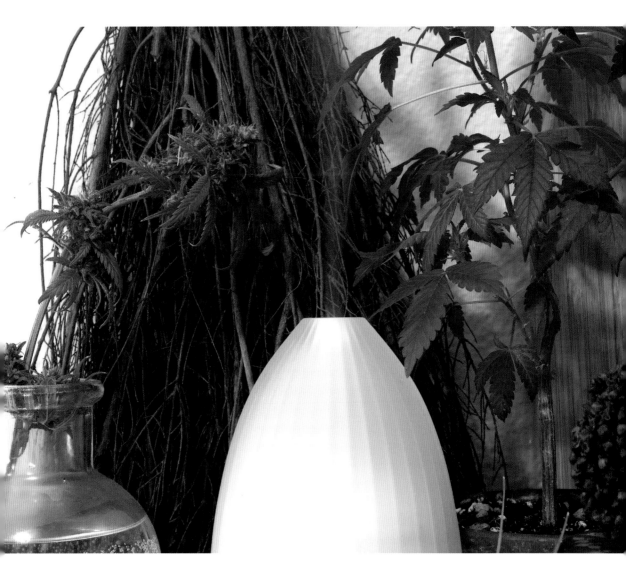

CHAPTER THREE

ESSENTIAL OIL BLEND RECIPES

These essential oil blend recipes were developed to stimulate your imagination about what's possible when you're working with essential oils, CBD, and hemp. In chapters 6 and 7, you will be introduced to spa recipes such as roll-ons, massage oils, creams, salves, CBD aromatherapy, bath fizz, and salts that will call for essential oils to create the entourage effect by pairing terpenes with your favorite CBD and hemp products.

To begin, you can try the technique of using a water-based essential oil diffuser and adding your favorite essential oil blend recipe along with 3 to 5 drops of your favorite water-soluble CBD extract and diffusing into your environment. This is a method of microdosing CBD, and it's a great way to experiment with these recipes before trying them in other spa recipes, such as massage oil or bath salts. Diffusing these recipes first allows you to test and familiarize yourself with the effects of various terpenes.

Mindful

An invigorating blend featuring limonene and caryophyllene.
Motivation and focus for meditation and tasks.
Suggestions for use | diffused, roll-on, room spray

3 parts or single drops cloves
2 parts or single drops lemon
2 parts or single drops bergamot (bergapten-free bergamot essential oil is preferred)

Energetic

A stimulating blend featuring limonene, caryophyllene, cedrol, and camphene.
Banish sluggishness and begin your day fully awakened.
Suggestions for use | diffused, roll-on, room spray, bath salts

2 parts or single drops grapefruit
2 parts or single drops cypress leaf
1 part or single drop black pepper

Release and Relieve

A stress-release blend featuring zingiberene, bisabolene, linalool, and myrcene.
Soothing relief anytime.
Suggestions for use | diffused, salve, lotion, bath salt

4 parts or single drops ginger
2 parts or single drops lavender
1 part or single drop basil

Soul

An enlightening blend featuring pinene, myrcene, terpineol, and pinocamphone.
Purifying for the mind and soul.
Suggestions for use | diffused, salve, roll-on, room spray, bath salt

4 parts or single drops frankincense
3 parts or single drops juniper berry
2 parts or single drops hyssop

The Opening

An inspiring blend featuring carvone, myrcene, and cineole.
A veritable fountain of creativity when you need it the most.
Suggestions for use | diffused, roll-on, room spray, bath salt

3 parts or single drops eucalyptus
2 parts or single drops spearmint
2 parts or single drops basil

Holy Anointing

A spiritual blend featuring curzerene, cinnamaldehyde, humulene, and eugenol.
Based on the original formula described in the Old Testament.
Suggestions for use | diffused, massage oil, salve

3 parts or single drops myrrh
2 parts or single drops cinnamon
2 parts or single drops cannabis

Sacred Heart Cleanse

A heart chakra cleanse blend featuring thujone, pinene, camphor, geraniol, and nerolidol.
Great for clearing negativity and enhancing euphoria.
Suggestions for use | diffused, salve, roll-on, room spray, bath salt

4 parts or single drops frankincense
2 parts or single drops sage
2 parts or single drops rose

Rest and Refresh

A cooling blend featuring limonene, cineole, pinene, and menthol.
When rest requires a refreshing aroma to open breathing and soothe the heat of a fever.
Suggestions for use | diffused, roll-on, room spray, bath salt

3 parts or single drops rosemary
2 parts or single drops lemon
1 part or single drop peppermint

Healer's Balm

A warming blend of caryophyllene, curzerene, humulene, and eugenol.
Anti-inflammatory for deep healing and pain-relief applications.
Suggestions for use | diffused, salve, roll-on, lotion, massage oil, bath salt

4 parts or single drops copaiba
2 parts or single drops myrrh
1 part or single drop cloves

Pure Romance

A flirtatious floral blend of limonene, geraniol, myrcene, and farnesene.
This is a luscious blend for romantic massage and temple rubs.
Suggestions for use | diffused, roll-on, massage oil, room spray, bath salt

2 parts or single drops geranium
2 parts or single drops ylang ylang
2 parts or single drops sweet orange

Busy Day

A hardworking blend of limonene, cineole, pinene, and thymol.
Great to diffuse in the car while sitting in commute traffic to soothe stress and increase alertness.
Suggestions for use | diffused, room spray, bath salt

3 parts or single drops orange
2 parts or single drops rosemary
1 part or single drop thyme

Haint Blue

A ghost-busting blend of chamazulene, pinene, nerol, sabinene, and limonene. Haint blue, the traditional southern color to chase away hauntings, is interpreted in this essential oil blend.
The blue oil that chases away the blues!
Suggestions for use | diffused, roll-on, room spray, bath salt

4 parts or single drops frankincense
2 parts or single drops blue tansy
1 part or single drop melissa (lemon balm)

Midnight Sun

A Nordic blend featuring anethole, pinene, and myrcene.

These essential oils come from traditional Nordic herbals and are paired with hemp—diffuse or make a thick salve to uplift, purify, and soothe.

Suggestions for use | diffused, roll-on, salve, room spray, bath salt

2 parts or single drops fennel
2 parts or single drops juniper berry
2 parts or single drops fir needle

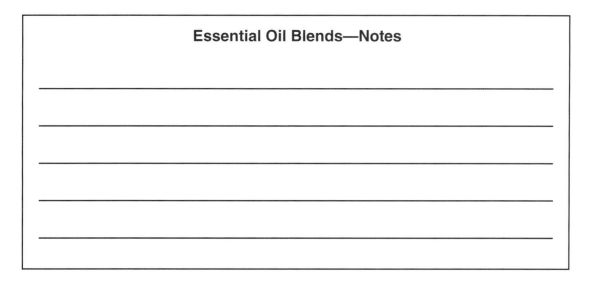

Essential Oil Blends—Notes

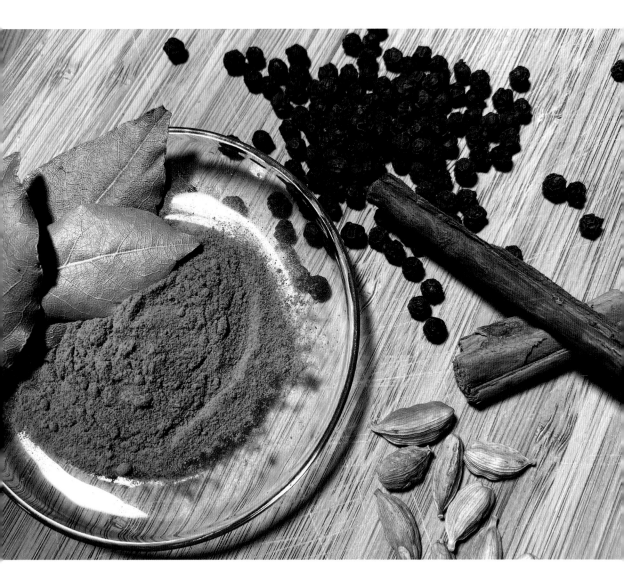

CHAPTER FOUR

SPICES AND AROMATICS BLEND RECIPES

Included in this chapter are whole aromatic herb and spice blend recipes and some suggested uses when pairing with your favorite CBD or hemp product. In chapter 8 (page 129), you will find culinary recipes using whole aromatics rich in terpene content paired with both CBD and hemp. But you don't have to limit your use to culinary only—whole aromatics also make beautiful spa products like salves and bath salts. You'll find suggestions for using some whole aromatic spices and herbs in chapters 6 and 7, too!

Harvest Spice

A traditional fall blend featuring caryophyllene, cinnamaldehyde, eugenol, zingiberene, and myrcene. It's one interpretation of "pumpkin spice," which has many different interpretations, and is generally used as a seasonal fall and winter spice.

It's warming and soothing as well as being invigorating for a time of year when some of us are more sluggish.

Suggestions for use | beverages, sweets, and pomades for aromatherapy

3 parts cinnamon
1 part cloves
1 part ginger
1 part allspice
1 part cardamom

Floral Refuge

A fresh floral blend featuring caryophyllene, geraniol, nerolidol, limonene, and safranal. Create beautiful moods and uplifted spirits with this unique all-floral blend.

Suggestions for use | tea, tisanes, candy, and in bath salts for spa

4 parts citron zest (Buddah's Hand or Etrog)
3 parts rose petals or buds
1 part cassia buds
(20 threads) saffron for every ½ cup or 100 grams of the other parts combined

Spices and Aromatic Blends—Notes

_____

_____

_____

_____

_____

Citrus Grove

A bright blend featuring limonene, myrcene, and nerolidol.

Refreshing and revitalizing.

Suggestions for use | tisane; sweets; savory foods like noodles, soup, dipping sauces; bath salts for spa time

1 part lemon zest
1 part orange zest
1 part kaffir leaves

Emerald Seasoning Blend

A soothing blend featuring myrcene, carvone, linalool, and terpineol.

Inspired by the cannabis-growing region of the Emerald Triangle in California, this blend is mellow and cheerful.

Suggestions for use | savory foods like salad dressing blends, vegan bean dishes, and seasoning for steamed vegetables

3 parts lemon thyme
2 parts spearmint
2 parts basil
2 parts marjoram

Spices and Aromatic Blends—Notes

_____

_____

_____

_____

Berry Wonderland

A potentiating blend featuring anethole, myrcene, geraniol, and linalool.
Myrcene will be the most notable terpene in this blend and is known for its ability to potentiate cannabinoids like CBD.

Suggestions for use | candy, sweets, tea, and tisane

3 parts blackberry
3 parts mango
1 part star anise

Mulling Blend

A warming anti-inflammatory blend featuring caryophyllene, cinnamaldehyde, linalool, eugenol, and myrcene.
This blend uses whole spices exclusively for infusions.

Suggestions for use | hot apple cider, hot pomegranate cider, and hot pear cider infusion, mulled wine and mead, tea, and tisane

3 parts cinnamon sticks
2 parts whole allspice berries
2 parts orange peels
1 part white peppercorn

Spices and Aromatic Blends—Notes

_____

_____

_____

_____

Jerk on Fire

A Caribbean blend featuring caryophyllene, myrcene, limonene, zingiberene, and cultivars of the hottest peppers on earth! Invigorating, anti-inflammatory, and pain-relieving, this blend works well in many savory dishes.

Suggestions for use | savory salad dressing, all-purpose seasoning for meat and vegetables, popcorn or popped sorghum seasoning

4 parts allspice
3 parts thyme
3 parts ginger
2 parts lemon zest
1 part habanero or ghost pepper

Golden Blend

An anti-inflammatory super-blend featuring turmerone, zingiberene, caryophyllene. Golden blend is one of the most versatile spice blends in the world that will lend a healing vibe to many preparations, both edible and spa.

Suggestions for use | beverages like "golden milk," tea, tisane, sweets, savory dishes, and spa preparations like pain-relieving salves

4 parts turmeric
3 parts ginger
1 part black pepper

Spices and Aromatic Blends—Notes

_____

_____

_____

_____

_____

Hot and Cold

A surprising blend featuring cooling carvone, and bisabolol terpenes paired with the heat of capsicum.

This blend is effective for pain related to nerve conditions when formulated as a spa preparation.

Suggestions for use | tisane, and spa applications like salve, lotion, balm

1 part cayenne pepper
1 part chamomile
1 part spearmint

Middle Ages Blend

A European purification blend featuring caryophyllene, limonene, pinene, and myrcene. This blend will clear and purify the environment.

Suggested uses | potpourri sachet for bed pillows, pomade for inhalation, and spa applications such as bath salts

1 part cloves
1 part orange zest
1 part thyme
1 part rosemary

Spices and Aromatic Blends—Notes

_____

_____

_____

_____

The Awakening

A motivational blend featuring caryophyllene, cinnamaldehyde, and limonene.

A great way to start the day as a blend for breakfast tea.

Suggestions for use | tea, tisane, and spa applications like bath salts

4 parts lemon zest
1 part mixed peppercorn
1 part cinnamon

Gingerbread House

An interpretation of a traditional blend featuring zingiberene, caryophyllene, myrcene, and cinnamaldehyde.

This blend is warming, soothing, and anti-inflammatory.

Suggestions for use | sweets like cookies, cakes, bars, and as an infusion for black tea

4 parts ginger
1 part cloves
1 part nutmeg
1 part cinnamon

Pretty Pepper Blend

A stimulating Asian-inspired blend featuring the terpenes caryophyllene and nerolidol paired with capsicum and the unique compound of hydroxy alpha sanshool.

This blend is floral, spicy, green, and slightly numbing and will lend an interesting effect and complex flavor.

Suggestions for use | savory dishes like seasoning for mochi, salad dressing, seasoning blend vegetables, tofu, or fish

2 parts white peppercorn
2 parts Sichuan pepper
1 part whole shishito pepper

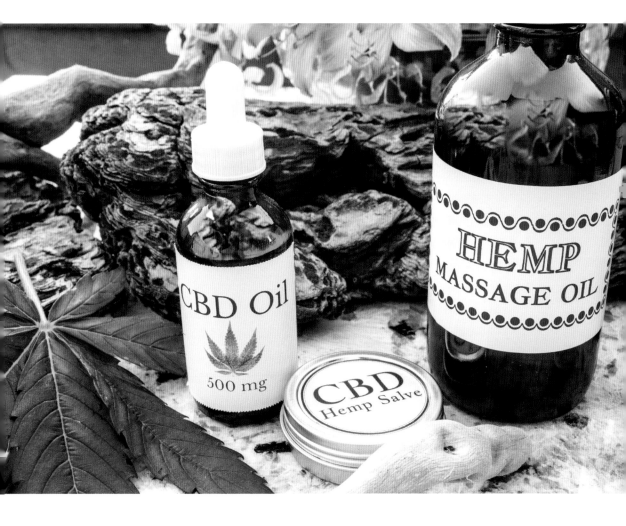

CHAPTER FIVE

AROMATHERAPY AND SPA WITH HEMP AND CBD

In this chapter, we will elevate our hemp and CBD experience with aromatherapy techniques and spa recipes.

The Art of Cannabis Aromatherapy

There are many aromatherapeutic techniques to enjoy both CBD and hemp, and these range from essential oils infused with CBD, which can be diffused into a room for microdosing, to aromatherapy roll-ons with CBD or hemp seed oil for temples or pressure points, and personal spritzers for quick aromatherapy anytime you need it. Best of all, these recipes and techniques are incredibly easy to use with your favorite CBD oil, CBD extract, or hemp seed oil.

This chapter builds on the concepts that you learned in chapter 2 about terpenes, CBD, hemp, and the entourage effect, and references many of the terpene blends you learned about in chapters 3 and 4. If you've tried your hand experimenting with essential oils and herbs from those chapters, use the planner pages for building an aromatherapy kit to use with any recipe or application.

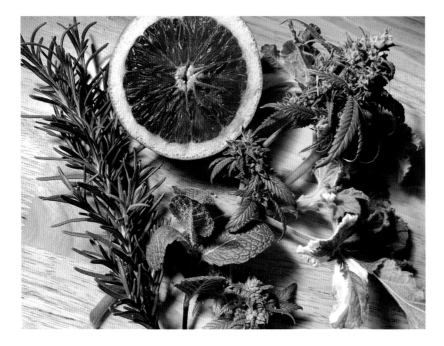

Cannabis Flower Essence Complementary

In chapter 1, we explored the concept of flower essences and how these are produced as commercial products that you can use in any aromatherapy, edible, or spa recipe as a complementary enhancement. Cannabis flower essence can also be made at home—but only if you have access to fresh, living hemp or cannabis flowers. Flower essences of any kind cannot be made with cured or dried plant material. That said, if you are not in a location where you can legally grow or obtain fresh, live hemp or cannabis flowers, you can purchase a tincture of a single hemp or cannabis flower essence and use this along with other kinds of fresh, living flowers to create your own unique flower essence blends. This chapter includes the recipe technique for making cannabis flower essence with fresh, live hemp

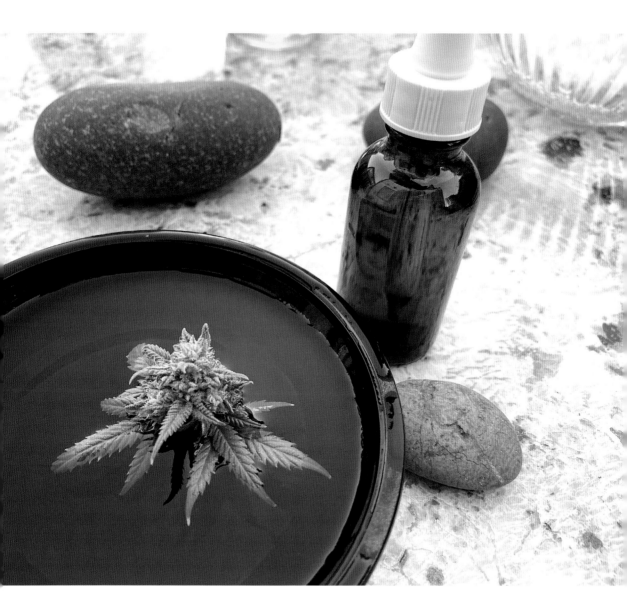

Aromatherapy and Spa with Hemp and CBD ✳ 57

or cannabis flowers, and the information about making cannabis flower essence blends using a commercial single hemp or cannabis flower essence blend and other fresh live flowers of your choice.

Cannabis flower essences are formulations based on the classical method and philosophy of flower essence creation and use. Bach Flower Essences are probably the best-known commercial product and classical method of creating flower essences, but the art of flower essence creation is not limited to only one "correct" method. Rather, due to the subjective and spiritual nature of the philosophy of flower essences, there are many different interpretations of this herbal art form. Generally speaking, the art form adheres to a simple framework from which many possibilities can emerge.

- Flower essence contains only vibrational or spiritual imprints of flowers—it **does not contain any botanical material**. This makes every flower essence safe for all people and animals.
- Flower essences are not homeopathy—although there may seem to be similarities, flower essences are based on spiritual principles. Flower essences do not cure or treat physical diseases, though traditional practice with Bach flower essences suggests use for addressing underlying spiritual or subjective aspects of illness. Flower essences are safe to use with any science-based medical treatment or any other complementary remedy without risk of incompatibility.
- Cannabis flower essences, like all flower essence formulations, contain only the vibrational or spiritual imprints and energetics of the cannabis flower and companion flowers, and none of the botanical material or cannabinoids like CBD or THC. This makes commercial cannabis flower essences legal in every location—although production will be limited to locations where cannabis has legal status.

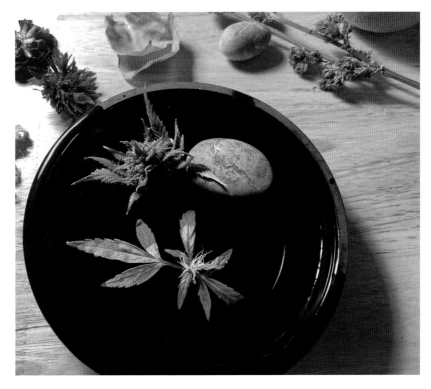

Cannabis Flower Essence Recipe

1. In a glass bowl (MIRON violet glass is suggested for best results), cut several fresh hemp or cannabis flowers that "speak" to you and float them in cold, sterilized spring water or rainwater. If you are using a MIRON glass charging bowl, place the lid on the bowl and set it in direct sun for 1 to 2 hours to create the vibrationally infused part of the mother tincture. If you are using a regular glass bowl, cover this with a very loose mesh that will let the sunlight pass through before placing outside in the sun.

(Continued on page 60)

2. Select the spirits you would like to use to preserve the mother tincture. The traditional spirit used to tincture flower essence is brandy—but you can use any clear 100+ proof spirit that you prefer with a neutral flavor and fragrance, such as white rum, moonshine, or grappa.
3. Prepare, boil/sterilize, and dry an amber or MIRON glass mother tincture bottle. Remove the bowl from the sun and strain the flowers from the water using a clean cheesecloth and strainer into the mother tincture bottle until it is half full. Fill the rest with the high-proof spirit you have selected, secure the lid, and shake. This is your mother tincture, of which you can make successive tinctures of cannabis flower essence.
4. Label your mother tincture with the vibrational qualities you have intuitively discovered from working with these flowers.
5. Use your mother tincture to make successive tinctures by adding one or two drops of the mother tincture to a new bottle and filling it with half sterilized spring water or rainwater and half high-proof spirits.

How to Make a Blended Cannabis Flower Essence

1. Select your favorite cannabis flower essence brand or your own hand-made cannabis flower essence for this recipe.
2. Following steps 1 through 5 of the Essence Recipe above, select fresh, living flowers to blend with your cannabis flower essence and use the same technique described for making cannabis flower essence to make any other flower essence.
3. Bottle and label your flower essence with the vibrational qualities you have intuitively discovered by working with the flowers.
4. In a clean, new amber or MIRON glass tincture bottle, add a drop or two of the cannabis flower essence along with drops of the other flower essences you have created to make a unique flower essence with the vibrational qualities that you desire. Fill halfway with sterilized spring

water or rainwater, and top off the bottle with the high-proof spirit you have chosen.

5. Affix the dropper top and shake. Label the bottle with the flower essences you have used and what the vibrational qualities are of this blend. Use as desired. Suggested shelf life is one year, but it may remain potent for longer.

How to Use Cannabis Flower Essences

Cannabis flower essences, being vibrational, spiritual, or meditation tools, can be used in almost any way you desire. Typically, one or two drops are used at a time to energize a larger volume of water or other consumables. Using a drop of cannabis flower essence along with spring water and essential oils in an aromatherapy diffuser is one favored method of many who enjoy flower essences. Try one drop of the essence in bathwater or to energize a larger volume of water, such as a hot tub. If you are preparing a glass beverage dispenser of water infused with fruit, flowers, or herbs, you can include a drop of cannabis flower essence to add pleasant vibrational effects. Adding a drop of the essence to a cup of tea for meditation purposes is also another way to work with cannabis flower essence. Like other kinds of flower essence, only one or two drops are needed at any one time and for any purpose. Furthermore, a tincture of the essence can be stretched further by adding a drop or two to spring water and then using an equal amount of brandy or other high-proof alcohol to preserve it and create an entirely new tincture.

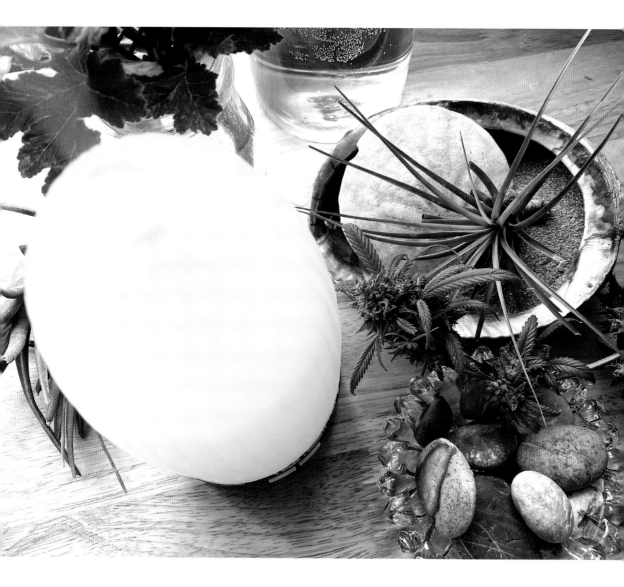

CBD: Enhancing Your Experience with Diffusion Techniques and Tools

Microdosing CBD is a popular way to enjoy nuanced benefits of CBD—and aromatherapy is the perfect vehicle for microdosing. *Microdosing* is defined as using extremely small amounts of a cannabinoid like CBD exclusively for a subtle and nuanced experience. Diffusion and spritzing are two of the simplest ways to enjoy using microdosed CBD.

For diffusion, you will need a standard water diffuser for essential oils. You can purchase essential oils already infused with CBD and use several drops in your diffuser with distilled or spring water, or you can purchase essential oils and water-soluble CBD extract and use a few drops in your diffuser along with the essential oils. Diffuse this in any space you wish to enhance with aromatherapy and CBD. Additionally, your diffuser is an excellent tool to enjoy the vibrational benefits of cannabis flower essences, and these pair perfectly with essential oils and CBD—simply add a drop of cannabis flower essence or any flower essence blend to your diffuser.

Spritzing is another microdosing aromatherapy technique that can be used directly on the skin and hair or to spritz your personal space for an immediate aromatherapy pick-me-up. These are portable and can be customized with all of the attributes you desire in personal CBD aromatherapy and are detailed in the following chapter.

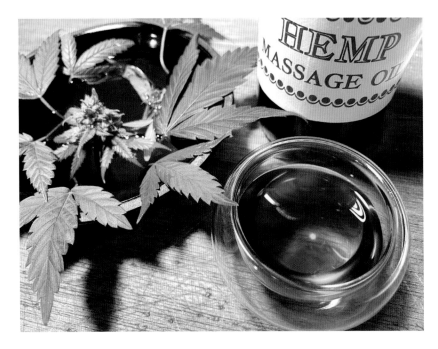

Hemp and CBD Spa and Beauty

Working with Hemp Seed Oil in Skin Care

Making handmade spa and beauty using hemp seed oil is similar to working with hemp seed oil for culinary recipes. Most hemp seed oil sold at retail and grocery stores is cold-pressed raw and unrefined—which is used primarily for culinary recipes, but also works great for spa and beauty. Unrefined hemp seed oil will have a more neutral fragrance and color than unrefined—most commercial spa and beauty products that contain hemp seed oil, such as lotions, contain refined hemp seed oil. The reason for this is that commercial spa products require a longer shelf life and more stability, and refined hemp seed oil is more stable in a variety of environmental and manufacturing conditions than unrefined hemp seed oil.

Furthermore, hemp seed oil, unrefined or refined, does not contain any cannabinoids, including CBD or THC.

Whether you will be working with unrefined culinary-grade hemp seed oil or refined oil, the same rules apply:

- Hemp seed oil should be kept in refrigeration until you are ready to use it in recipes.
- Processing temperatures should never exceed 250° F (121° C) and heat should only be applied for very short periods of time, and only when necessary, such as to blend hemp seed oil with other solid fats and waxes that have been melted to create a salve, massage oil, or other spa products.
- Hemp seed oil products where hemp seed oil is the base or a primary ingredient have shorter shelf lives than other types of oil or wax, such as jojoba or MCT (fractionated coconut oil). For this reason, it is useful to include an antioxidant such as rosemary, like we have done for our roll-on recipes in the following chapter. For the recipes in chapter 7, rosemary antioxidant is also preferred antioxidant ingredient.

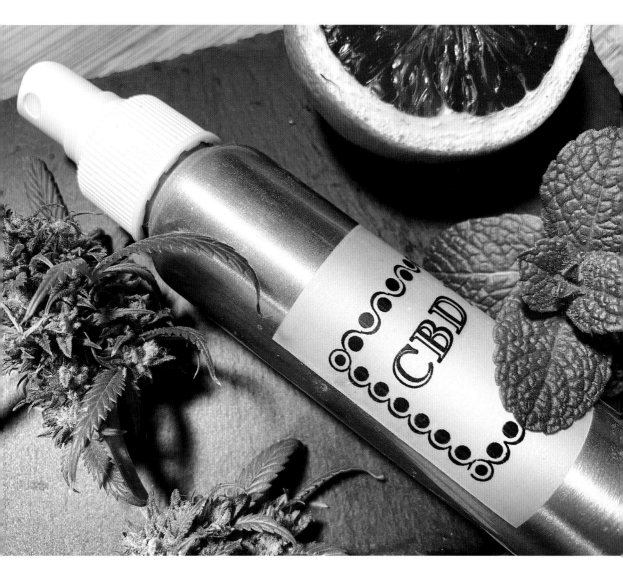

CHAPTER SIX

CBD AND HEMP SEED OIL SPRITZ AND ROLL-ON RECIPES

Ingredients:

1 ounce (30 ml) 100+ proof clear, neutral spirits such as white rum, moonshine, grappa, or brandy

1 suggested spritzer blend (to follow), or one that you formulate using your favorite essential oil brands and the worksheet included on page 69

1 teaspoon (5 ml) or less of your favorite water-soluble CBD extract brand

3 ounces (90 ml) of sterilized distilled water (boil to sterilize or use bottled)

1 drop or more of your favorite cannabis flower essence or blend, or any other flower essence you desire (optional)

Quick or Portable CBD Aromatherapy with Spritzing

To make CBD-infused spritzers, you will use water-soluble CBD extract, essential oils, a high-proof spirit, distilled water, and cannabis flower essence as an optional ingredient. These spritzers should be stored in a glass or aluminum bottle with a sprayer—do not store in plastic, as essential oils can sometimes degrade plastic.

Spritzer Base

Makes one 4-ounce (120 ml) personal spritzer

Instructions:

1. Boil to sterilize and dry a glass or aluminum bottle. Use high-proof spirit to sanitize the sprayer and allow it to air dry.
2. Add the high-proof alcohol, the essential oil blend you have selected, the water-soluble CBD extract, distilled water, and the optional flower essence. Affix the lid and shake vigorously before spraying. Shake each time before use. Shelf life is up to one year.
3. Spritz your personal space or directly on the body—do not spray directly into face or eyes.

Cleansing

This blend will clear and refresh your personal space, mind, and body.

7 drops rosemary
3 drops eucalyptus
3 drops lemon

Dreaming

Use this blend to open the imagination while awake or dreaming.

7 drops frankincense
3 drops lavender
2 drops clove
1 drop cinnamon

Uplifting

This blend is a mood-enhancer that can be used to brighten the mood and uplift the vibrations of your personal space.

6 drops lemon
3 drops orange
2 drops grapefruit
2 drops peppermint

Relaxing

A lovely blend for relaxation at the end of the day.

6 drops lavender
4 drops cedarwood
2 drops lemongrass

Your Personal CBD Aromatherapy Spritz Blend Worksheet

Use this worksheet to formulate your own CBD aromatherapy spritz blends based on what you've learned about pairing terpenes (essential oils) with your favorite CBD extracts in chapter 2.

Spritzer Blend Name	CBD Extract Selection (include brand and milligrams)

From most to least, record each essential oil and the number of drops per 4-ounce (120 ml) spritzer.

Essential Oil #1	Essential Oil #1	Essential Oil #1	Essential Oil #1	Essential Oil #1

Note the therapeutic and vibrational effects of your blend and any recipe additions such as flower essence.

Therapeutic and Vibrational Notes

Spritzer Blend Name	CBD Extract Selection (include brand and milligrams)

From most to least, record each essential oil and the number of drops per 4-ounce (120 ml) spritzer.

Essential Oil #1	Essential Oil #1	Essential Oil #1	Essential Oil #1	Essential Oil #1

Note the therapeutic and vibrational effects of your blend and any recipe additions such as flower essence.

Therapeutic and Vibrational Notes

Spritzer Blend Name	CBD Extract Selection (include brand and milligrams)

From most to least, record each essential oil and the number of drops per 4-ounce (120 ml) spritzer.

Essential Oil #1	Essential Oil #1	Essential Oil #1	Essential Oil #1	Essential Oil #1

Note the therapeutic and vibrational effects of your blend and any recipe additions such as flower essence.

Therapeutic and Vibrational Notes

Spritzer Blend Name	CBD Extract Selection (include brand and milligrams)

From most to least, record each essential oil and the number of drops per 4-ounce (120 ml) spritzer.

Essential Oil #1	Essential Oil #1	Essential Oil #1	Essential Oil #1	Essential Oil #1

Note the therapeutic and vibrational effects of your blend and any recipe additions such as flower essence.

Therapeutic and Vibrational Notes

Spritzer Blend Name	CBD Extract Selection (include brand and milligrams)

From most to least, record each essential oil and the number of drops per 4-ounce (120 ml) spritzer.

Essential Oil #1	Essential Oil #1	Essential Oil #1	Essential Oil #1	Essential Oil #1

Note the therapeutic and vibrational effects of your blend and any recipe additions such as flower essence.

Therapeutic and Vibrational Notes

Spritzer Blend Name	CBD Extract Selection (include brand and milligrams)

From most to least, record each essential oil and the number of drops per 4-ounce (120 ml) spritzer.

Essential Oil #1	Essential Oil #1	Essential Oil #1	Essential Oil #1	Essential Oil #1

Note the therapeutic and vibrational effects of your blend and any recipe additions such as flower essence.

Therapeutic and Vibrational Notes

Spritzer Blend Name	CBD Extract Selection (include brand and milligrams)

From most to least, record each essential oil and the number of drops per 4-ounce (120 ml) spritzer.

Essential Oil #1	Essential Oil #1	Essential Oil #1	Essential Oil #1	Essential Oil #1

Note the therapeutic and vibrational effects of your blend and any recipe additions such as flower essence.

Therapeutic and Vibrational Notes

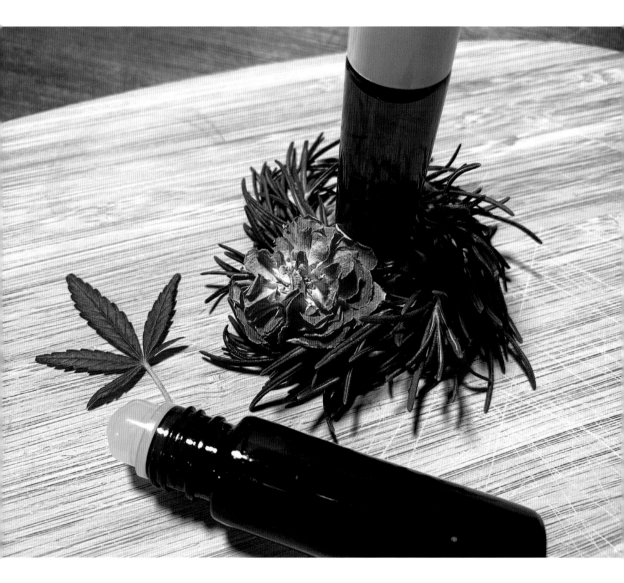

CBD and Hemp Seed Oil Aromatherapy Roll-On Recipes

Roll-ons are a neat and convenient way to enjoy the therapeutic benefits of both CBD oil and hemp seed oil. These recipes take no more than five minutes to make and allow you dozens of options to choose from when formulating with your favorite oils.

These can be used in a variety of ways, including as a temple rub or on pressure points like acupressure points. They can also be used as a joint rub on knees or even smaller joints like fingers or wrists. Roll-ons should not be used near the eyes, mouth, or mucous membranes to avoid sensitivity. Test in a small area first, such as your arm, before applying elsewhere on the body for best results.

Formulate with Hemp Seed Oil

Hemp seed oil is a very delicate oil that can become rancid when exposed to normal shelf conditions for an extended period of time. To extend the shelf life of hemp seed oil aromatherapy roll-ons, and other spa recipes that include hemp seed oil, we will pair with another oil (called a carrier oil), such as rice bran oil, jojoba oil, or MCT (fractionated coconut oil). Jojoba is a favorite of many for these roll-ons and has the longest shelf life. The addition of a few drops of a low-cost specialty ingredient called rosemary antioxidant, which comes from rosemary, can also help extend the life of a hemp seed oil–based roll on. Use these within 6 months for best results. This recipe does not contain cannabinoids like CBD or THC.

Makes 1 roller bottle (amber glass is preferred) 1 or 2 ounces (30–60ml)

Instructions:

1. Boil/sterilize a glass roller bottle, and soak the roller ball top in alcohol to sanitize. Allow to completely dry before filling.
2. Add the hemp seed oil first, then the essential oils, and top with the carrier oil you have selected, along with the rosemary antioxidant. Affix the roller top and screw on the lid.
3. Shake vigorously to thoroughly combine all the ingredients. Your roll-on is now ready to use.

Ingredients:

1 part hemp seed oil
1 suggested roller blends (to follow), or one that you formulate using your favorite essential oil brands and the worksheet included on page 82
1 part jojoba, rice bran, or MCT (fractionated coconut oil)
0.5 milliliters rosemary antioxidant

Formulate with CBD Oil

For this recipe, you will select your favorite CBD oil and pair it with a carrier oil and an essential oil blend to create a roll-on that has the benefits of both CBD and terpenes. You can use this roll-on the same way you use the roll-on made with hemp seed oil: as a temple rub, at pressure points, or as a joint rub. Use within 6 months for best results.

Makes 1 roller bottle (amber glass is preferred) 1 or 2 ounces (30–60ml)

Ingredients:

1 part carrier oil (suggested oils for maximum absorption and shelf life are jojoba, olive, rice bran, camellia seed, meadowfoam seed, or MCT (fractionated coconut oil)

1 teaspoon (5 ml) or less of your favorite CBD oil

1 suggested roller blend (to follow), or one you formulate using your favorite essential oil brands and the worksheet included on page 82

Instructions:

1. Boil/sterilize a glass roller bottle, and soak the roller ball top in alcohol to sanitize. Allow to completely dry before beginning.
2. Add the carrier oil first, then the CBD oil and essential oils. Affix the roller top and screw on the lid.
3. Shake vigorously to thoroughly combine all the ingredients. Your roll-on is now ready to use.

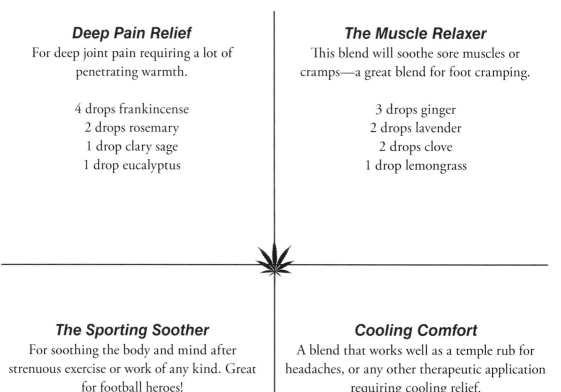

Deep Pain Relief

For deep joint pain requiring a lot of penetrating warmth.

4 drops frankincense
2 drops rosemary
1 drop clary sage
1 drop eucalyptus

The Muscle Relaxer

This blend will soothe sore muscles or cramps—a great blend for foot cramping.

3 drops ginger
2 drops lavender
2 drops clove
1 drop lemongrass

The Sporting Soother

For soothing the body and mind after strenuous exercise or work of any kind. Great for football heroes!

5 drops copaiba
2 drops clove
2 drops ginger
1 drop clary sage

Cooling Comfort

A blend that works well as a temple rub for headaches, or any other therapeutic application requiring cooling relief.

2 drops peppermint
1 drop geranium
1 drop lemon
1 drop chamomile

Temple Rub

A gentle temple rub for motivation and focus
when you need it the most.

5 drops frankincense
2 drops black pepper
2 drops copaiba

Pressure-Point Remedy

This pressure-point remedy
uses resinous oils from ancient
remedies renowned for their therapeutic effects.
Use at the desired pressure points on your body.

3 drops frankincense
2 drops myrrh
1 drop copal
1 drop Atlas cedarwood

Gentle Lullaby

This blend promotes gentle and restful
sleep at nighttime or for that well-deserved
daytime nap.

4 drops chamomile
3 drops frankincense
1 drop lavender

Tranquil Moment

The perfect blend of meditation—
try this in a roll-on for yoga time
or anytime you need a tranquil moment.

2 drops spearmint
2 drops thyme
2 drops lavender
2 drops frankincense

Your Personal CBD and Hemp Seed Oil Aromatherapy Roll-On Blend Worksheet

Use this worksheet to formulate your own CBD and hemp seed oil aromatherapy roll-on blends based on what you've learned about pairing terpenes (essential oils) with your favorite CBD oil or hemp seed oil in chapter 2.

Roll-On Blend Name	CBD Oil Selection (include brand and milligrams) or hemp seed oil

From most to least, record each essential oil and the number of drops per 1–2 ounce (30–60 ml) roll-on.

Essential Oil #1	Essential Oil #1	Essential Oil #1	Essential Oil #1	Essential Oil #1

Note the therapeutic and vibrational effects of your blend.

Therapeutic and Vibrational Notes

Roll-On Blend Name	CBD Oil Selection (include brand and milligrams) or hemp seed oil

From most to least, record each essential oil and the number of drops per 1–2 ounce (30–60 ml) roll-on.

Essential Oil #1	Essential Oil #1	Essential Oil #1	Essential Oil #1	Essential Oil #1

Note the therapeutic and vibrational effects of your blend.

Therapeutic and Vibrational Notes

Roll-On Blend Name	CBD Oil Selection (include brand and milligrams) or hemp seed oil

From most to least, record each essential oil and the number of drops per 1–2 ounce (30–60 ml) roll-on.

Essential Oil #1	Essential Oil #1	Essential Oil #1	Essential Oil #1	Essential Oil #1

Note the therapeutic and vibrational effects of your blend.

Therapeutic and Vibrational Notes

Roll-On Blend Name	CBD Oil Selection (include brand and milligrams) or hemp seed oil

From most to least, record each essential oil and the number of drops per 1–2 ounce (30–60 ml) roll-on.

Essential Oil #1	Essential Oil #1	Essential Oil #1	Essential Oil #1	Essential Oil #1

Note the therapeutic and vibrational effects of your blend.

Therapeutic and Vibrational Notes

Roll-On Blend Name	CBD Oil Selection (include brand and milligrams) or hemp seed oil

From most to least, record each essential oil and the number of drops per 1–2 ounce (30–60 ml) roll-on.

Essential Oil #1	Essential Oil #1	Essential Oil #1	Essential Oil #1	Essential Oil #1

Note the therapeutic and vibrational effects of your blend.

Therapeutic and Vibrational Notes

Roll-On Blend Name	CBD Oil Selection (include brand and milligrams) or hemp seed oil

From most to least, record each essential oil and the number of drops per 1–2 ounce (30–60 ml) roll-on.

Essential Oil #1	Essential Oil #1	Essential Oil #1	Essential Oil #1	Essential Oil #1

Note the therapeutic and vibrational effects of your blend.

Therapeutic and Vibrational Notes

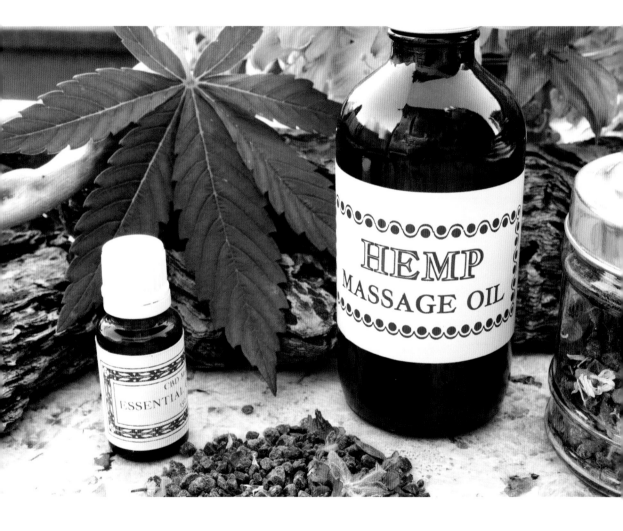

CHAPTER SEVEN

HEMP-INFUSED AND CBD-INFUSED SPA RECIPES

Hemp-Infused Spa Recipes

The following recipes can be made with either raw and unrefined hemp seed oil or refined hemp seed oil—you can even experiment with both and select your favorite. You are encouraged to experiment with these recipes, using what you have learned about terpene pairing with hemp and CBD. Additionally, these recipes can be formulated free of terpenes to create fragrance-free recipes, which are preferred by many skin professionals, especially for those with skin sensitivities and allergies.

Hemp seed oil is noncomedogenic (will not clog pores or encourage acne) and is extremely nourishing for the skin and hair—it is a superior moisturizing and skin-softening ingredient for all skin types.

Massage Master Oil

This recipe can make any amount of massage oil that you desire.

This is a silky massage oil that will glide over the skin for any kind of massage technique. It can be customized by selecting an essential oil blend with the terpene content you desire—or formulated fragrance-free.

Instructions:

1. Boil/sterilize any glass or aluminum bottle that will hold your massage oil. Sanitize a pump dispenser lid with alcohol. Allow to dry completely.
2. Add the hemp seed oil and jojoba oil and combine thoroughly.
3. Depending on the amount of hemp seed oil and jojoba oil you have combined, add the requisite amount of rosemary antioxidant and thoroughly combine.
4. At this point, if you wish to have a fragrance-free massage oil, you can affix the pump or lid and begin using the oil. If you have decided to pair terpenes with your massage oil, add the requisite essential oils depending on the amount of massage oil you have made, and shake to combine.
5. Prepare a pan of water with hot tap water and place the bottle of oil into the pan of water and gently warm it to thoroughly infuse all ingredients. After the water has cooled, remove the bottle and shake it again. Use this oil within 6 months for best results. Keep away from heat and light to maintain freshness.

Ingredients:

1 part hemp seed oil
1 part jojoba oil
1 milliliter rosemary antioxidant per 4 ounces (120 ml) of massage oil
10 drops, or less, any terpene (essential oil) blend from chapter 2 or 3, per 4 ounces (120 ml) of massage oil

After–Bath Body–Conditioning Oil

An after-bath hemp-infused oil that is lightly fragranced, refreshing, and moisturizing without being greasy or heavy—this oil is easy to make and contains essential oils with terpenes of pinene and linalool as an invigorating entourage for hemp. You can make this oil fragrance-free with the same great benefits by omitting the terpene content (essential oils).

Makes 8 ounces or 240 ml of body oil

Ingredients:

¾ cup (180 ml) sweet almond oil
¼ cup (60 ml) culinary hemp seed oil
1 milliliter rosemary antioxidant
Terpene (essential oil) blend (optional):
    5 drops of french lavender essential oil
    5 drops of spruce, fir, or pine essential oil

Instructions:

1. Boil/sterilize any glass or aluminum bottle that will hold your body oil. Sanitize a pump dispenser lid with alcohol. Allow to dry completely.
2. Combine the sweet almond oil, hemp seed oil, and rosemary antioxidant. At this point, if you wish to have a fragrance-free body oil, you can affix the pump or lid and begin using the oil. If you have decided to pair terpenes with your massage oil, add the essential oils and shake to combine.
3. Prepare a pan of water with hot tap water and place the bottle of oil into the pan of water and gently warm it to thoroughly infuse all ingredients. After the water has cooled, remove the bottle and shake it again. Use this oil within 6 months for best results. Keep away from heat and light to maintain freshness.

How to use:

After bathing, pour out a small coin-sized amount of the oil into your hand. Apply evenly to the skin. The oil, when applied evenly in small amounts, should absorb quickly immediately after bathing.

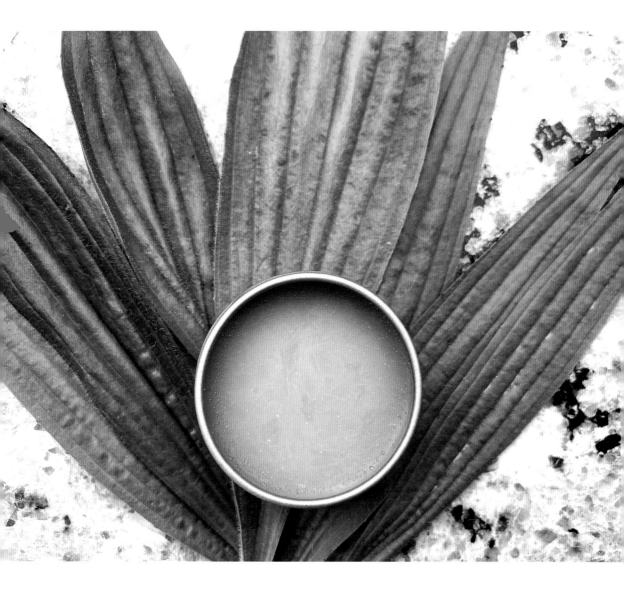

Garden and Kitchen Salve

A beautiful salve for hardworking hands—this salve is beneficial for gardeners, chefs, or as an all-around great kitchen salve. This recipe uses the novel ingredient (and common backyard weed) plantain paired with hemp seed oil to create a healing and soothing salve for dry, overworked hands and small scrapes and bumps.

Plantain (*Plantago major* and *Plantago lanceolata*) can be found everywhere, but the best place to collect clean plantain leaves will be your own backyard or any pristine open field. Plantain leaves can also be purchased from any bulk herbal supplier, as well, if you prefer. Making this salve with plantain leaves that you have foraged is very satisfying and makes the best-quality salve.

Makes about 5 ounces (150 ml) salve

Ingredients:

1 small handful plantain leaves (about 5–10 leaves)
⅓ cup (80 ml) coconut oil
3 tablespoons (45 ml) beeswax or candelilla wax
2 tablespoons (30 ml) hemp seed oil
2 milliliters rosemary antioxidant

Instructions:

1. If you are using fresh plantain leaves, wash them thoroughly and then lay them out on a paper towel overnight to dry and wilt. If you are using dried leaves from an herbal apothecary supplier, skip this step.
2. Boil/sterilize the glass or aluminum jar you will be using for your salve and allow to dry thoroughly.
3. In a slow cooker or pan on the stove, melt the coconut oil on the lowest setting. Once the coconut oil is melted and hot (approximately 180° F or 82° C), add the plantain leaves and turn off the heat. Allow the plantain leaves to infuse into the warm coconut oil for an hour.
4. After infusion, turn on the heat so that the coconut oil is very liquid and hot (approximately 180° F or 82° C). Turn off the heat, and strain the plantain leaves from the coconut oil. Add the wax to the hot oil and melt to combine thoroughly.

(Continued on page 94)

5. Add the hemp seed oil and rosemary antioxidant to the mixture while it is still warm and liquid, and stir to combine thoroughly.
6. Pour into the salve jar you have prepared and allow this to sit on the counter for about 20 minutes. Transfer to the freezer and allow the salve to completely solidify, about 30 minutes. This step will prevent the grainy texture that is common in salve left to fully solidify at room temperature.
7. Remove from the freezer. Your salve is ready for use and will be shelf-stable at room temperature. Allow to sit on the counter for 30 minutes before affixing the lids. Store away from heat sources in your kitchen. Use within 6 months for best results.

Easy Makeup Remover Ointment

In the mid-twentieth century, petroleum jelly had a special place on every woman's vanity for daily use—and one of the most common uses of petroleum jelly was to remove makeup at the end of the day. This beauty ointment is efficient for removing makeup but is made with plant-based ingredients instead of petroleum-based ingredients and has a similar texture and ease of use as petroleum jelly. Best of all, it's made with noncomedogenic ingredients like hemp seed oil that will not clog pores or encourage breakouts.

This makeup remover ointment does not have any terpene addition. For best results, it is suggested as a fragrance-free recipe.

Makes about 8 ounces (235 ml) ointment

Ingredients:
⅓ cup (80 ml) shea butter
⅔ cup (160 ml) hemp
    seed oil
1 milliliter rosemary
    antioxidant

Instructions:
1. Boil/sterilize a glass jar and allow this to thoroughly dry.
2. In a slow cooker or a pan on the stove, gently melt the shea butter. After melted and fully liquid, turn off the heat and add the hemp seed oil and rosemary antioxidant, and stir until thoroughly combined.
3. Pour the liquid ointment into the glass jar and allow it to remain on the counter for about 20 minutes before transferring to the refrigerator to cool for 20 minutes. This will ensure the finished ointment does not have a grainy texture after it has cooled.
4. Remove from the refrigerator. The ointment will be somewhat solidified at this point, but as it warms to room temperature, it will become a softer ointment. Affix the lid and store on your vanity for ease of use as a makeup remover. Use within 6 months for best results.

How to use:
Scoop the ointment with your fingers or a flat cosmetic spoon implement and generously apply to the entire face. Use a soft cloth or tissue to wipe away the ointment and makeup. Wash your face as you normally would.

Hemp Beautiful Salve

Salve is a very popular natural health product today—but did you know that salves can also serve as a beauty product in a similar way to moisturizers? This beauty salve is a must-have for your bag as a quick beauty pick-me-up any time of day. It can be used on cheeks, lips, and hands.

This recipe is a bit more complex, but well worth the effort. It contains hemp seed oil and ingredients that absorb quickly and are not greasy. If you are not able to obtain authentic rose essential oil, you may substitute rose geranium essential oil. Authentic rose essential oil is a luxury ingredient that will give the best results and you will only need one drop. Some reliable essential oil brands sell sample sizes in this amount for a few dollars if you do not want to spend $100 or more on several milliliters of this rare and precious essential oil.

Makes 5.5 ounces (160 ml) of salve, which can be split between several small tins

Instructions:

1. Boil/sterilize a glass jar and/or smaller metal tins and allow these to thoroughly dry.
2. In a slow cooker or a pan on the stove, gently melt the shea butter, camellia seed oil or meadowfoam seed oil, and wax together. After melted and fully liquid, turn off the heat and add the hemp seed oil, rosemary antioxidant, and essential oils, and stir until thoroughly combined.
3. Working quickly, pour the liquid salve into the glass jar and/or salve tins and allow them to remain on the counter for about 20 minutes before transferring to the freezer to solidify completely and cool for 20 minutes. This will ensure that the finished ointment does not have a grainy texture after it has cooled.
4. Remove from the freezer. The salve will be solid and ready for use. Allow to sit on the counter for 30 minutes before affixing the lids. The salve is now shelf-stable and should be stored away from heat. Use within 6 months for best results.

Ingredients:

¼ cup (60 ml) shea butter

2 teaspoons (10 ml) camellia seed oil or meadowfoam seed oil

2 tablespoons (30 ml) beeswax or candelilla wax

¼ cup (60 ml) hemp seed oil

1 milliliter rosemary antioxidant

1 drop rose essential oil or rose geranium essential oil

1 drop spearmint essential oil

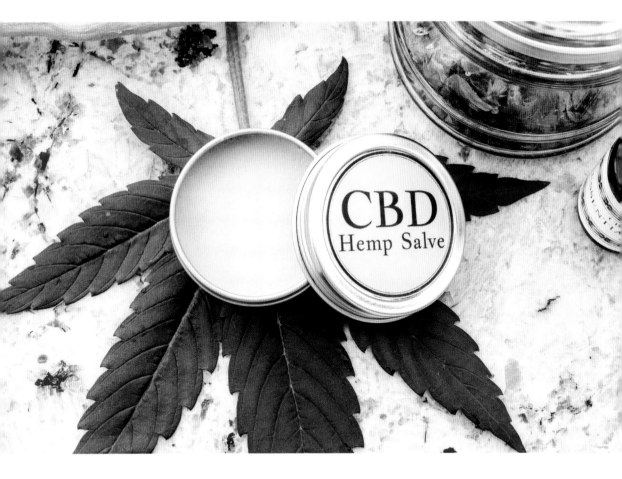

Easy Hemp Vanilla Bean Body Butter

A body butter than smells so sweet you'll want to taste it! And that's okay, because this body butter is made with all edible ingredients. The decadence of cocoa and vanilla bean paired with unrefined hemp seed oil creates the most luxurious and delicious body butter you'll ever use. You can purchase all of the ingredients at your local natural foods grocer.

Makes 8 ounces (240 ml) body butter

Instructions:

1. Boil/sterilize a glass jar and allow this to thoroughly dry.
2. In a slow cooker or a pan on the stove, gently melt the cocoa butter. After the cocoa butter melts, add the whole vanilla bean, and hold the cocoa butter and vanilla bean on the lowest warm setting for 1 hour so that the vanilla bean fully infuses into the cocoa butter.
3. Turn off the heat and remove the vanilla bean from the cocoa butter. Pour the infused cocoa butter into a bowl, add the hemp seed oil and rosemary antioxidant, and stir until thoroughly combined. Allow to sit on the counter for 10 minutes.
4. Cover the bowl and put it into the refrigerator for 10 minutes. Take the bowl out of the refrigerator and, using a hand mixer or blender, vigorously whip the mixture. Place the bowl back into the refrigerator for 10 more minutes, remove from the refrigerator, and vigorously whip again. Repeat this step several times until the body butter has gone from a liquid to a creamy whipped butter.
5. Spoon the body butter into the glass jar you have prepared. Affix the lid. It should be stored in a cool area, such as a cabinet or drawer away from heat sources, or in the refrigerator to maintain the buttery texture. If the butter melts, it can be cooled and whipped again to revitalize the texture. Use within 6 months for best results.

Ingredients:

¾ cup (180 ml) cocoa butter, culinary grade
1 vanilla bean, sliced open
¼ cup (60 ml) unrefined culinary grade hemp seed oil
1 milliliter rosemary antioxidant

Hemp Hair Oil and Conditioning Treatment

Hemp seed oil is one of the most nourishing and moisturizing oils for the hair and scalp and can be applied neat. For best results, it is suggested to make the hair oil with refined hemp seed oil. Unrefined culinary-grade hemp seed oil can also be used but will have a shorter shelf life. This oil can be used as a preconditioning treatment before shampooing or after shampoo on damp hair for best results.

Makes any amount of hair oil you desire, but small batches are best

Ingredients:

1 part hemp seed oil, refined (for best results) or unrefined culinary grade

1 milliliter rosemary antioxidant per 4 ounces (120 ml) hemp seed oil

Terpene blend (essential oils) beneficial for scalp and hair, per 4 ounces (120 ml) hemp seed oil (optional):

    2 drops clary sage
    2 drops thyme
    2 drops cedarwood

Instructions:

1. Boil/sterilize a glass or aluminum bottle to use to store your hemp hair oil. Sanitize the pump or lid with alcohol. Allow to dry completely.
2. Fill the bottle with hemp seed oil and add the requisite amount of rosemary antioxidant and optional essential oil terpene blend. Affix the lid or pump.
3. Prepare a bowl of hot tap water and gently warm the oil in the bottle for 20 minutes. Remove the bottle from the water and shake. The hair oil is now ready for use. Store in a cool area or in the refrigerator. Use within 6 months for best results.

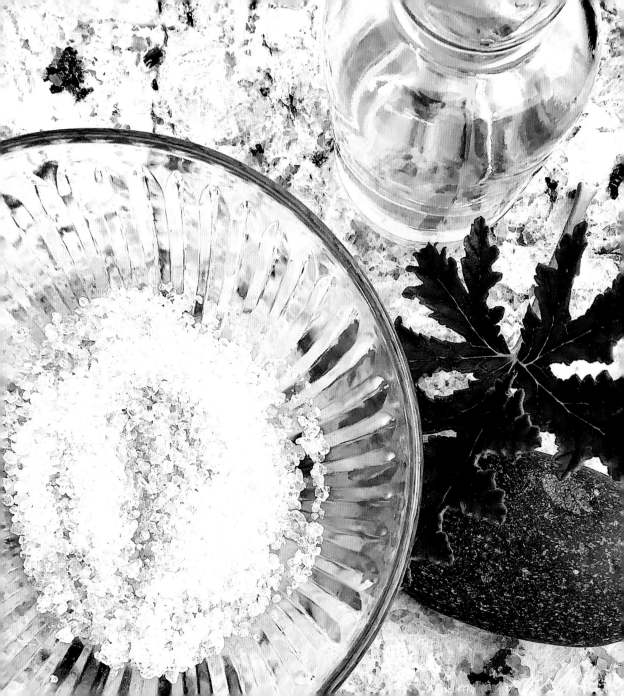

Beautiful Hands Hemp Soak

Moisturize and soften hands as part of your manicure regime with this hot oil soak recipe and technique. This Mediterranean-inspired formulation will exfoliate dry skin and moisturize nails and cuticles. Get beautiful hands anytime!

Makes as much oil soak as you desire

Ingredients:

2 parts olive oil
1 part hemp seed oil
1 milliliter rosemary antioxidant per 4 ounces (120 ml) soaking oil
Terpene (essential oil) blend for hands and nails, per 4 ounces (120 ml) soaking oil (optional):
   3 drops rosemary essential oil
   1 drop lavender essential oil
   1 drop lemon essential oil
Coarse sea salt or Dead Sea salt (for filling the soaking bowl)

Instructions:

To prepare the hand soak oil:

1. Boil/sterilize a glass or aluminum bottle to use to store your hand soak oil. Sanitize the pump or lid with alcohol. Allow to dry completely.
2. Fill the bottle with the olive oil and hemp seed oil and add the requisite amount of rosemary antioxidant and optional essential oil terpene blend. Affix the lid or pump.
3. Prepare a bowl of very hot tap water and place the bottle in the hot water, allowing it to gently warm the oils inside for 20 minutes. Remove the bottle from the water and shake. The hand soak oil is now ready for use. Store in a cool area or in the refrigerator. Use within 6 months for best results.

How to prepare a hand soak session:

1. Fill a glass bowl (approximately cereal bowl–sized) about halfway with coarse sea salt or Dead Sea salt. The salt should be deep enough to cover the hands to about the knuckles when hands are submerged in the salt.
2. Put the salt in a warm oven for 10 minutes or microwave for 5 seconds until it is very warm but not too hot for the skin. Stir in 1 tablespoon (15 milliliters) or a little more of the hand soak oil into the warm salt and stir until combined thoroughly.

3. Before soaking your hands, clean and dry them. Plunge the hands into the warm salt and oil and massage the hands and nails with the warm oil and salt for several minutes until the mixture cools completely. This is very effective for warming arthritic finger joints prior to the warm water soak.

4. Prepare some warm water and pour the salt and oil mixture into the warm water and soak the hands up to the wrists for 10 minutes. Massage the oil into the hands, and then remove from the water and dry with a clean towel. The water can now be discarded.

Exfoliating Sugar Scrub

Sugar scrubs are a delightful way to experience the skin benefits of hemp seed oil. This scrub will revitalize and polish the skin, sweeping away dead skin cells and revealing beautiful moisturized skin—ideal for exfoliating the skin before a bath or shower!

Makes a little more than 8 ounces (300 g) of sugar scrub

Ingredients:

3 tablespoons (45 ml) of coconut oil

3 tablespoons (45 ml) of hemp seed oil

1 milliliter rosemary antioxidant

Terpene (essential oil) blend (optional):

    6 drops of sweet orange oil

    3 drops of lavender oil

1 cup (250 g) coarse turbinado sugar

Instructions:

1. Boil/sterilize a glass jar and allow it to thoroughly dry before beginning.
2. In a small dish or pan, gently melt the coconut oil. After the coconut oil is melted, remove from the heat and add the hemp seed oil, rosemary antioxidant, and optional essential oil blend, and stir until thoroughly combined. Allow the oil to sit on the counter for 15 minutes.
3. Add the sugar to the pan and stir in the oils. Spoon the mixture into the clean jar you have prepared and place in the refrigerator for 25 minutes.
4. Remove from the refrigerator and stir again. The sugar scrub is ready to use. Affix the lid and store in a cool area or in the refrigerator. Use within 6 months for best results.

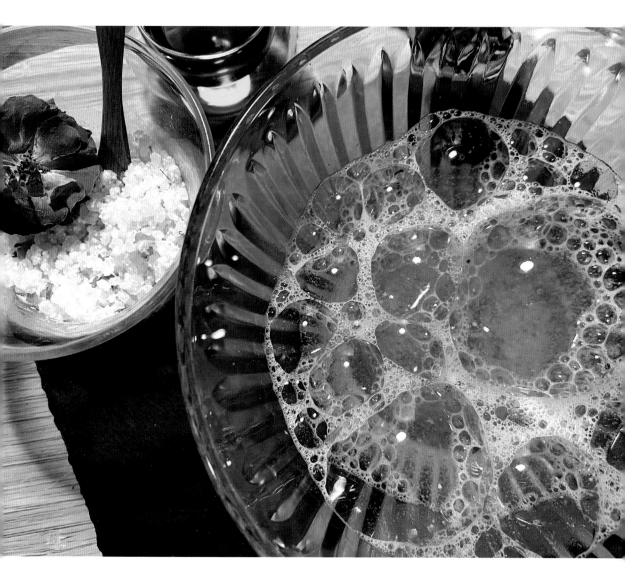

Moisturizing Hemp Bath Salts

Create a spa bath that will relax you and make your skin silky soft with a little fizz! Experience the therapeutic effects of hemp seed oil and terpenes. This bath salt can be customized to any terpene (essential oil) blend that you have explored in chapter 2.

Makes any amount of bath salts you prefer

Ingredients:

4 parts sea salt or pink Himalayan salt
2 parts baking soda
1 part citric acid
10 drops terpene (essential oil) blend of your choice from chapter 2 (page 23) per 2 cups (600 g) finished bath salt
1 tablespoon (15 ml) hemp seed oil per 2 cups (600 g) finished bath salt

Instructions:

1. Boil/sterilize the glass jar you will use to store your bath salts and allow this to dry completely.
2. In a bowl, thoroughly combine the salt, baking soda, and citric acid.
3. Add the essential oil blend to the hemp seed oil and thoroughly combine. Add this to the salt a little at a time while stirring to slowly combine and evenly distribute.
4. Spoon the finished salt into the jar and tightly affix the lid to keep out moisture. Use within 6 months for best results.

How to use:

Use about a handful or a little more for larger tubs. This bath salt works best in warmer water temperatures for the full experience with the terpene content of the bath.

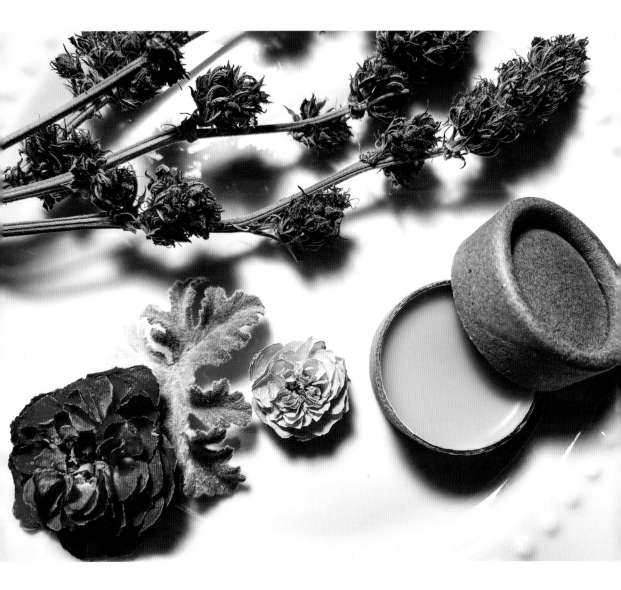

CBD-Infused Spa Recipes

The following spa recipes incorporate your favorite CBD oil and extracts—and these recipes will allow you to adjust them to the dosages of CBD that you desire.

A word about dosing for spa:

The recipes have a recommended amount of CBD oil or extract. This is based on incorporation with the other ingredients; CBD oil and CBD extracts come in many different milligram strengths and suggested doses made by the manufacturer. For example, 1 teaspoon (5 milliliters) of CBD oil with 50 milligrams versus the same amount with 10 milligrams. You can use the milligram dosages that you desire, but the actual amount of oil or extract should not exceed the suggested volume in the recipe so that the oil or extract can be successfully infused into the recipe. You may, however, use less than the suggested volume if you desire.

Hemp Seed Oil and CBD Therapeutic Oil Soak for Nails

Pair the beneficial moisturizing effects of hemp seed oil with CBD for a therapeutic nail soak that will soften cuticles and skin and also reduce inflammation.

Makes any amount of oil soak that you desire

Instructions:

1. Boil/sterilize the glass (amber glass is preferred) or aluminum bottle you will be using for your oil, and dry completely.
2. Combine the rice bran oil and hemp seed oil along with the requisite amounts of rosemary extract and CBD oil in the bottle, affix the lid, and shake thoroughly.
3. Prepare a bowl with hot tap water and allow the bottle of oil to gently warm for about 20 minutes. Shake again to ensure even distribution of all ingredients. Store away from heat and light. Use within 6 months for best results.

How to use:

Pour a little bit of the oil in a small shallow bowl and gently warm for 3 to 5 seconds in the microwave or in a pan with hot water. The oil should be comfortably warm to the touch. Hands should be very clean and dry before soaking the fingertips in the oil for 15 minutes. The oil can be reused several times, but do not pour back into the original bottle.

Ingredients:

2 parts rice bran oil
1 part hemp seed oil
2 milliliters rosemary extract per 1 cup (240 ml) oil soak
1 teaspoon (5 ml) or less of your favorite CBD oil per 1 cup (240 ml) oil soak

Everyday Healer Salve

Have you been curious about the soothing benefits of CBD salve, but you've never tried it before? This basic salve recipe is a great way to experience a CBD topical because it's so easy to make with basic kitchen ingredients and versatile for many uses. Essential oils (terpenes) are optional—try it with your favorite blend of terpenes or fragrance-free.

Makes as much salve as you desire

Ingredients:

2 parts olive oil
1 part beeswax or candelilla wax
1 teaspoon (5 ml) or less of your favorite CBD oil per 4 ounces (120 ml) of salve
10 drops terpene (essential oil) blend of your choice from chapter 2 (page 23) per 4 ounces (120 ml) salve (optional)

Instructions:

1. Boil/sterilize a glass jar and/or smaller metal tins and allow these to thoroughly dry.
2. In a slow cooker or a pan on the stove, gently melt the olive oil and wax together. After melted and fully liquid, turn off the heat, add the CBD oil and essential oils, and stir until thoroughly combined.
3. Working quickly, pour the liquid salve into the glass jar and/or salve tins and allow them to remain on the counter for about 20 minutes before transferring to the freezer to solidify completely and cool for 20 minutes. This will ensure that the finished ointment does not have a grainy texture after it has cooled.
4. Remove from the freezer. The salve will be solid and ready for use. Allow to sit on the counter for 30 minutes before affixing the lids. The salve is now shelf-stable and should be stored away from heat. Use within 6 months for best results.

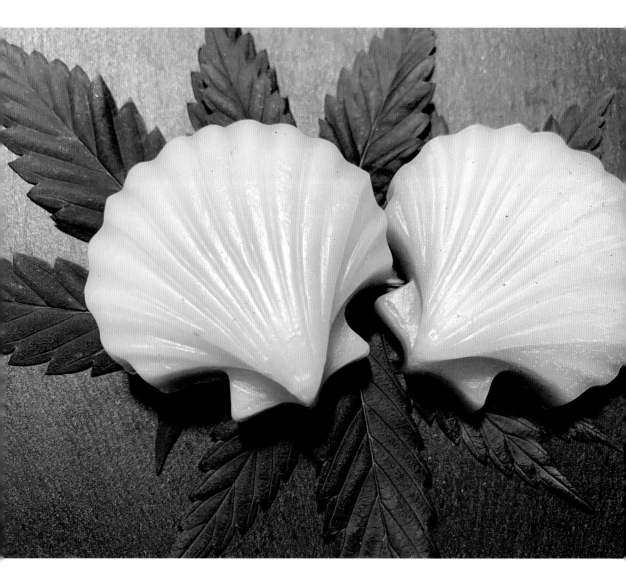

Everything Lotion Bars

Lotion bars are a great way to enjoy the benefits of your favorite CBD oil as a spa treatment. This simple recipe is easy to make and can be made with or without CBD. Wrap them in wax paper or parchment paper bags. These lotion bars are also a great gift idea, as they are portable and eliminate the need for packaging, such as plastic lotion bottles or other liquid containers. Perfect for the gift recipient who has never tried CBD!

Makes as many lotion bars as you desire

Ingredients:

1 part shea butter
1 part beeswax or candelilla wax
1 part hemp seed oil
1 milliliter rosemary antioxidant per 1 cup (240 ml) melted lotion bar liquid
2 teaspoons (10 ml) or less of your favorite CBD oil per 1 cup (240 ml) melted lotion bar liquid*
10 drops terpene (essential oil) blend of your choice from chapter 2 (page 23) per 1 cup (240 ml) of melted lotion bar liquid (optional)

omit if you would like to make hemp seed oil only

Instructions:

1. Prepare the molds you will be using for the lotion bars by cleaning and allowing to dry thoroughly. Prepare the wax paper or parchment bags by cutting the correct size to wrap your lotion bars along with ribbon or decorative twine. Set aside.

2. In a slow cooker or pan on the stove, gently melt the shea butter and wax until liquid.

3. Turn off the heat and then add the hemp seed oil, rosemary antioxidant, CBD oil, and/or essential oils. Thoroughly combine.

4. Working quickly, pour the mixture into molds. Allow these to remain on the counter for 15 minutes and then move to the freezer until solid, about 20 minutes. This freezer step will ensure the bars will have a smooth texture.

5. Remove from the freezer and pop from the molds onto a clean surface. You may now wrap the bars with the paper and twine or ribbon that you have prepared. Use within 6 months for best results.

Massage Candles

Massage candles are a unique way to enjoy the therapeutic spa benefits of CBD oil, and like lotion bars, they make a really nice gift for any occasion. You will need widemouthed heat-safe glass (such as canning jars) and zinc-free candle wicks along with a few pairs of wooden chopsticks to hold the wicks in place after the massage candle is poured.

Makes as many candles as you desire.

Instructions:

1. Boil/sterilize the glass jar you will use for your massage candle(s) and allow this to dry completely.
2. Drop the wick into each jar you have prepared and tie the top of the wick to a chopstick to stabilize it in the center of the jar as the wax is poured around it.
3. In a slow cooker or a pan on the stove, gently melt the mango seed butter, and stir in the olive oil. Turn off the heat and stir in the CBD oil and the optional essential oils.
4. Working quickly, pour the melted candle into the jar(s). Gently tap on the counter to release air bubbles. Allow to remain on the counter for 30 minutes. Transfer to the refrigerator for an hour to fully harden.
5. Remove from the refrigerator and cut the wick, leaving about 1 inch of wick on top of the candle. Affix the lid. The candle is ready for use. Use within 6 months for best results.

How to use:

Light the candle and allow an even pool of melted oil to form. Carefully pour a small amount of melted massage oil into the hands before applying the warm oil to the body. The candle will last longer if the pool of oil is allowed to even out before extinguishing the candle.

Ingredients:

4 parts mango seed butter
1 part olive oil
1 teaspoon (5 ml) or less of your favorite CBD oil per 1 cup (240 ml) of massage candle oil
10 drops terpene (essential oil) blend of your choice from chapter 2 (page 23) per 1 cup (240 ml) massage candle oil (optional)

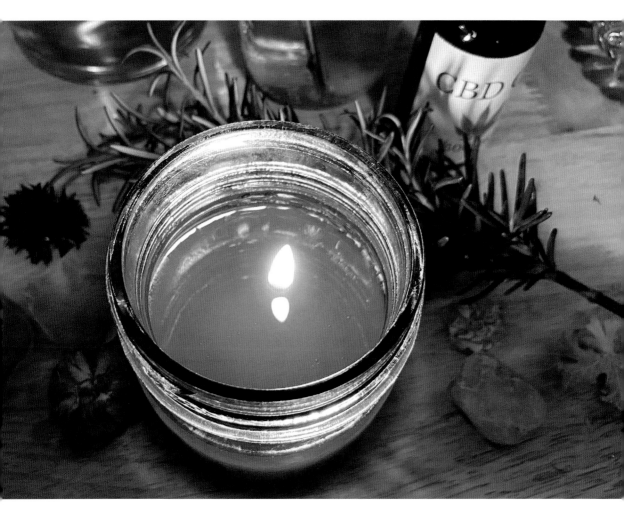

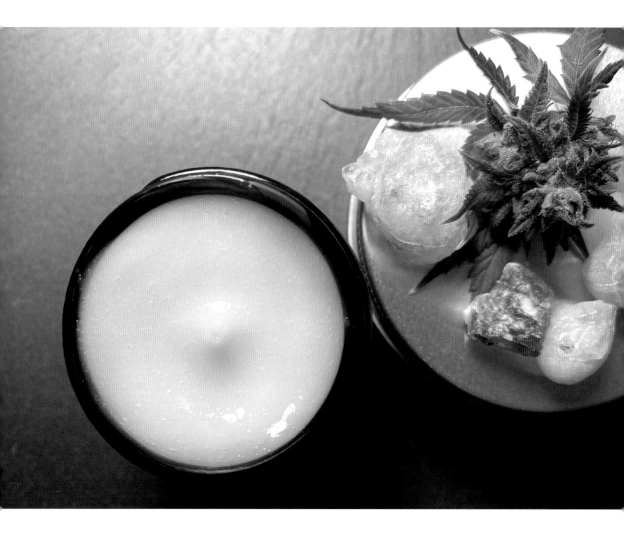

Frankincense Butter for Pain Relief

This recipe combines the powerful ingredients of frankincense resin with CBD oil to create a lush body butter with many therapeutic benefits. Anti-inflammatory, soothing, and healing—this body butter is unique, as it incorporates whole resin, not essential oil, to add the benefit of boswellic acid. Boswellic acid, the main active ingredient of frankincense, does not occur in the distilled essential oil. This body butter has a light frankincense fragrance that is more tenacious than the essential oil, as well.

Makes 8 ounces (240 ml) body butter

Ingredients:

¾ cup (180 ml) mango seed butter

¼ cup (60 ml) rice bran oil

1 tablespoon (15 g) frankincense resin

1 teaspoon (5 ml) or less of your favorite CBD oil

Instructions:

1. Boil/sterilize the glass jar you will use for your body butter and allow this to dry completely.
2. In a slow cooker or a pan on the stove, gently melt the mango seed butter, rice bran oil, and frankincense resin together on low until the frankincense resin has dissolved into the fats. Stir frequently. This step may take about 30 minutes. There will be some undissolved grains of the resin at the end—you can spoon these out. They are the water-soluble gum component in the resin.
3. Turn off the heat and pour the frankincense-infused oil into a bowl, add the CBD oil, and stir until thoroughly combined. Allow to sit on the counter for 10 minutes.
4. Cover the bowl and put it into the refrigerator for 10 minutes. Take the bowl out of the refrigerator and, using a hand mixer or blender, vigorously whip the mixture. Place the bowl back into the refrigerator for

(Continued on page 116)

10 more minutes, remove from the refrigerator, and vigorously whip again. Repeat this step several times until the body butter has gone from a liquid to a creamy, whipped butter.

5. Spoon the body butter into the glass jar you have prepared. Affix the lid. It should be stored in a cool area, such as a cabinet or drawer away from heat sources, or in the refrigerator to maintain the buttery texture. If the butter melts, it can be cooled and whipped again to revitalize the texture. Use within 6 months for best results.

Sports Recovery Massage Oil

A simple CBD massage oil that can be prepared in a snap and even made into a hard salve with only olive oil! This massage oil is deeply penetrating and will soothe sore muscles and joints after strenuous physical activity.

Makes any amount of massage oil you desire

Ingredients:

1 part olive oil
2 teaspoons (10 ml) or less of your favorite CBD oil per 1 cup (240 ml) massage oil
Terpene (essential oil) blend per 1 cup (240 ml) massage oil:
    3 drops rosemary essential oil
    3 drops peppermint essential oil
    3 drops pine essential oil

Instructions:

1. Boil/sterilize the glass jar or bottle you will use for your massage oil and allow this to dry completely.
2. In a bowl, combine the olive oil, CBD oil, and the essential oil blend. Pour into the glass jar or bottle you have prepared.
3. If you will be using the massage oil as a liquid, affix the pump lid to the bottle. The massage oil is ready for use.
4. If you would like to use this as a cool, solid massage oil, similar to a salve, affix the lid and place the jar into the freezer for about 30 minutes, until the oil fully solidifies. It can then be transferred to the refrigerator and will remain solid as long as it is kept in refrigeration. Use within 6 months for best results.

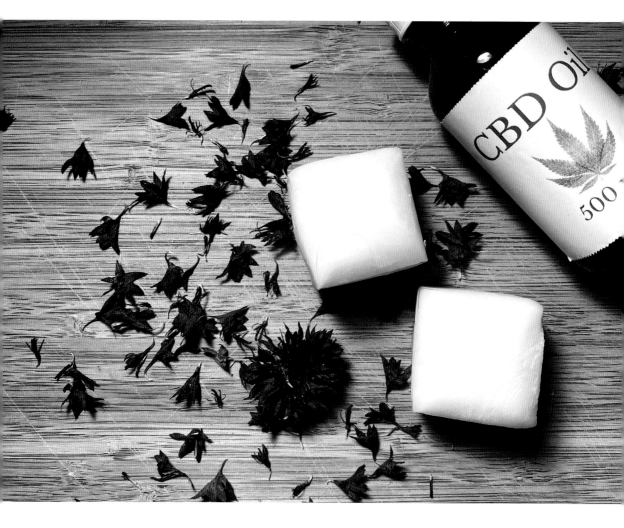

Fresh Cucumber Face and Body Lotion Cubes

A cooling, soothing, and moisturizing lotion cube that combines the therapeutic spa benefits of both hemp seed oil and CBD. This lotion cube is 100% free of preservatives, unlike most commercial bottled lotions, which must contain a preservative due to the water content. These lotion cubes are frozen into small cubes and used from the freezer as needed. You'll always have a fresh CBD-infused lotion cube anytime you need it—try these after a hot shower!

Makes about 12 small lotion cubes

Ingredients:

½ cup (120 ml) shea butter

2 tablespoons (30 ml) hemp seed oil

⅓ cup (80 ml) gel scraped from fresh aloe leaves*

1 peeled 5-inch (13-cm) piece cucumber

1 teaspoon (5 ml) or less of your favorite CBD oil

Do not use bottled aloe juice for this recipe.

Instructions:

1. Prepare the ice cube mold tray you would like to use for your lotion cubes by washing and drying thoroughly.
2. In a slow cooker or pan on the stove, melt the shea butter on low heat. Turn off the heat.
3. In a blender, add the hemp seed oil, the gel from the scraped aloe leaves, and the cucumber. Blend until smooth. Pour the mixture into a strainer lined with fine cheesecloth and press the liquid through the strainer into a bowl. Discard the fiber that remains after squeezing out all the liquid.
4. Pour the strained mixture into the warm oil and add the CBD oil. Using a hand blender, vigorously blend until creamy.
5. Working quickly, pour the mixture into ice cube trays and freeze immediately. Freeze until the lotion cubes are solid and pop out of the tray easily.
6. Pop the cubes out of the tray and put them into a sealed bag or container for storage in the freezer. Keep frozen and use within 3 months.

How to use:

Use these lotion cubes one at a time straight from the freezer directly on the skin.

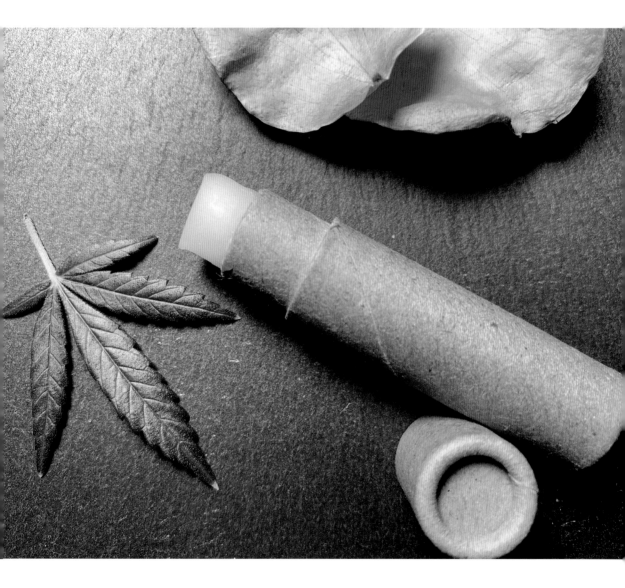

Tropical Beach Lip Balm

A beautiful CBD-infused lip balm that will moisturize and soothe dry and chapped lips. You'll love this sweet tropical lip balm that you can use every day. This lip balm pairs CBD with hemp seed oil to create the lip therapy you need right now!

Makes 2 ounces (60 ml) lip balm

Ingredients:

2 tablespoons (30 ml) beeswax or candelilla wax

1 tablespoon (15 ml) shea butter

1 tablespoon (15 ml) coconut oil

1 vanilla bean, sliced

2 teaspoons (10 ml) hemp seed oil

0.5 milliliters rosemary antioxidant

1 teaspoon (5 ml) or less of your favorite CBD oil

Terpene (essential oil) blend:
    1 drop of jasmine oil
    1 drop of spearmint oil

Instructions:

1. Clean and sanitize one or more lip balm tins with alcohol and allow to thoroughly dry.
2. In a slow cooker or pan on the stove, melt the wax, shea butter, and coconut oil on low heat. Add the vanilla bean and allow it to infuse into the oil on the lowest warm setting for 30 minutes.
3. Remove the vanilla bean from the warm oil and turn off the heat. Add the hemp seed oil, rosemary antioxidant, CBD oil, and the essential oil blend, and combine thoroughly.
4. Working quickly, pour the lip balm into the lip tin(s) or tube(s) and allow these to remain on the counter for 20 minutes. Move to the freezer and allow them to solidify completely. The freezer step will ensure the lip balm has a smooth texture after it solidifies completely.
5. Remove from the freezer and rest on the counter for 30 minutes before affixing the lid. Use within 6 months for best results.

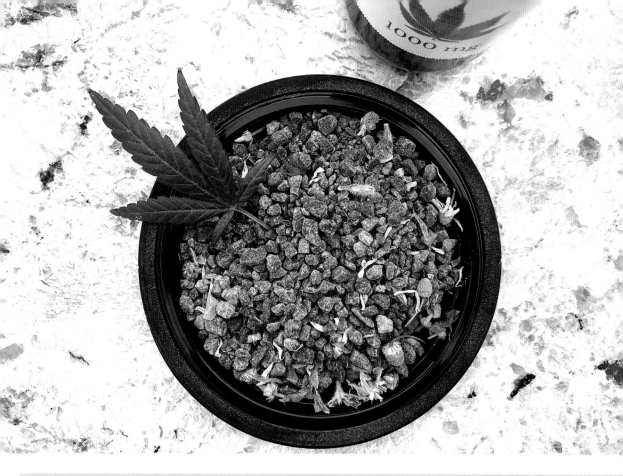

Used primarily as a culinary salt to add nuances of minerals and sulfur in Indian and Pakistani cuisine, black salt also has therapeutic uses, such as in spa formulations to create bathwater with similar characteristics to natural sulfur mineral springs. Black salt has a significant sulfur odor from the natural presence of sulfur in this mined rock salt, which was laid down by ancient seas millions of years ago. The most authentic black salt will be mined and packaged in its natural state, while cheaper black salt is sometimes created by taking Himalayan pink salt through a chemical process to create the presence of sulfur.

Sulfur is a naturally occurring element that has many benefits for the skin, especially for acne. Sulphur soaps and medicinal preparations have been used for centuries to balance the skin flora and purify and clear the skin as a remedy that is still in use today.

Black Salt Detox Bath Salts

A lesser known and highly mineralized variety of Himalayan pink salt is a salt known as *black salt*. This bath salt is paired with water-soluble CBD extract and some medicinal herbs to create a clean purification bath for troubled skin in need of special attention. Soak time will be 30 to 60 minutes to receive the most benefits. The bathwater should be as warm as you can tolerate to simulate the temperatures of natural sulfur hot springs.

Makes 1 pound (about 550 g) of bath salt*

Ingredients:

- ¼ cup (70 g) coarse rock Himalayan black salt
- 1¾ cups (490 g) coarse rock Pink Himalayan salt
- 10 drops rosemary essential oil
- 10 drops lemon essential oil
- 2 teaspoons (10 ml) or less of your favorite water-soluble CBD extract (select the highest concentration of CBD extract to use in this recipe)
- 1 well-rounded tablespoon (3 g) of mixed dried therapeutic terpene herbal blend like the Middle Ages Blend from chapter 2 (page 52)

Instructions:

1. Prepare a glass canning jar by boiling to sterilize and then drying completely.

2. In a glass or ceramic bowl, add the black salt, essential oils, and the CBD extract and thoroughly combine together until all of the salt is coated. Add the herbal blend and gently toss into the salt until evenly distributed.

3. Transfer the bath salt to the clean jar immediately. For best results, place a food-grade silicone moisture-absorbing pack in the jar to ensure the freshness of the bath salts, especially if this will be stored in the bathroom for convenience. These bath salts will have up to a one-year shelf life if they are kept dry and tightly closed.

---

*   This will equal approximately six average-sized baths, or three to four baths for large or jetted tubs. This bath will have a sulfur odor, which is normal. It is most beneficial not to shower immediately after taking this bath, but you can do so if you need to remove the odor of sulfur that may linger after this bath, which is similar to using a natural sulfur hot springs.

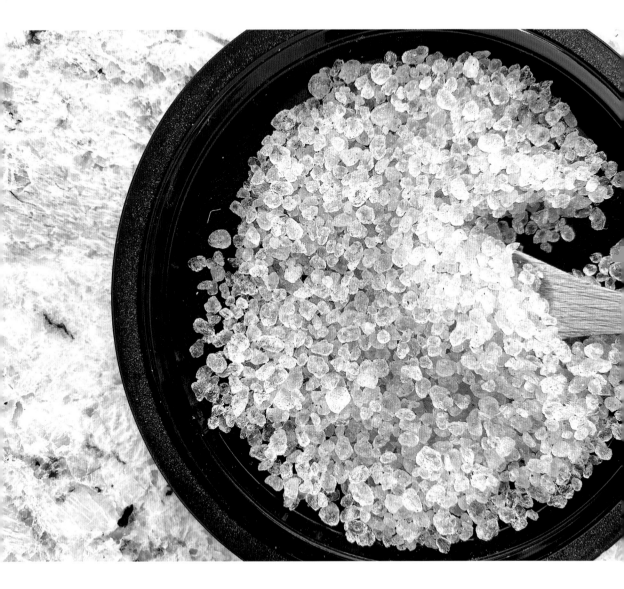

Pain-Relieving Bath Salts

Pain relief is one of the top reasons so many people are curious about CBD these days! CBD works best as a therapeutic ingredient for pain relief when it has an entourage of supporting elements, including terpenes, but also methods of use such as balneotherapy (bathing). This bath salt recipe uses Dead Sea salt for enhanced mineral content renowned for its therapeutic value. For ease of formulation, this bath salt uses your favorite water-soluble CBD extract, which will be evenly distributed throughout the bathwater. Use this bath salt in very warm water for best results.

Makes 1 pound (about 550 g) of bath salt*

Ingredients:

2 cups (550 g) coarse rock Dead Sea Salt

15 drops Healer's Balm terpene blend from chapter 2 (page 44) OR 5 drops clove oil and 10 drops eucalyptus oil

2 teaspoons (10 ml) or less of your favorite water-soluble CBD extract (select the highest concentration of CBD extract to use in this recipe)

1 well-rounded tablespoon (5 g) of powdered ginger

Instructions:

1. Prepare a glass canning jar by boiling to sterilize and then drying completely.
2. In a glass or ceramic bowl, add the Dead Sea salt, essential oils, and the CBD extract and thoroughly combine until all of the salt is coated. Add the powdered ginger to thoroughly coat the salt evenly.
3. Transfer the bath salt to the clean jar immediately. For best results, place a food-grade silica moisture-absorbing pack in the jar to ensure the freshness of the bath salts, especially if this will be stored in the bathroom for convenience. These bath salts will have up to one-year shelf life if they are kept dry and tightly closed.

---

* This will equal approximately six average-sized baths, or three to four baths for large or jetted tubs.

Rock-a-Bye Bath Salts

Epsom salt (magnesium sulfate), a common staple of medicinal baths found in most pharmacies and grocery stores, pairs with water-soluble CBD extract in this bath formulation designed for restful sleep and relief of nighttime leg cramps. This bath salt works best in a warm bath, but if you would like to relax in lukewarm or slightly cool water, dissolve the salts in warm water first and then run the bath until it reaches the temperature you prefer.

Makes 1 pound (about 550 g) of bath salt*

Instructions:

1. Prepare a glass canning jar by boiling to sterilize and then drying completely.
2. In a glass or ceramic bowl, add the Epsom salt, essential oils, and the CBD extract and thoroughly combine until all the salt is coated. Add the optional cornflower petals and gently toss into the salt until evenly distributed.
3. Transfer the bath salt to the clean jar immediately. For best results, place a food-grade silica moisture-absorbing pack in the jar to ensure the freshness of the bath salts, especially if this will be stored in the bathroom for convenience. These bath salts will have up to a one-year shelf life if they are kept dry and tightly closed.

Ingredients:

2 cups (550 g) coarse rock Epsom Salt

15 drops Release and Relieve terpene blend from chapter 2 (page 42) OR 5 drops lavender oil and 10 drops frankincense oil

2 teaspoons (10 ml) or less of your favorite water-soluble CBD extract (select the highest concentration of CBD extract to use in this recipe)

1 tablespoon (1 g) dried blue cornflower petals for a beautiful blue contrast in the salt and additional skin benefits (optional)

---

*   This will equal approximately six average-sized baths, or three to four baths for large or jetted tubs.

Purification Salt Scrub

Exfoliate, purify, and moisturize face and body with this outstanding CBD-infused salt scrub featuring antioxidant-rich matcha tea. Perfect for the end of the day to refresh the skin and revitalize the body. Try this scrub on elbows, knees, and feet!

Makes about 9 ounces (330 g) of salt scrub

Ingredients:

¾ cup (180 ml) coconut oil
1 teaspoon (5 ml) or less of your favorite CBD oil
1 tablespoon (5 g) matcha green tea
⅔ cup (185 g) fine grain sea salt

Instructions:

1. Boil/sterilize the glass jar you will use to store your salt scrub and allow this to dry completely.
2. Gently melt the coconut oil by resting the jar in a pan of hot water until it is liquid, and measure the correct amount of melted coconut oil before pouring into the bowl you will be mixing the salt scrub in.
3. Add the CBD oil and matcha green tea to the melted coconut oil and combine thoroughly.
4. Add the sea salt and combine thoroughly. Place the bowl in the refrigerator and allow the coconut oil to become thick. Take it out and stir again to evenly distribute the salt and other ingredients.
5. Spoon into the jar and affix the lid. Your salt scrub is ready to use. Use within 3 months for best results. The scrub should not come into contact with moisture in order to stay fresh.

How to use:

Scoop some out with dry fingers and use on the skin before a bath or shower.

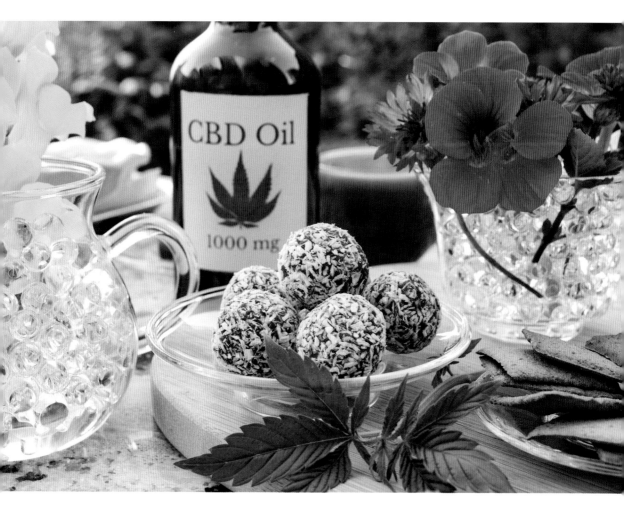

CHAPTER EIGHT

CANDY, BITES, AND BREWS: DELICIOUS AND FUN RECIPES

Easy, edible recipes with CBD, hemp, and your favorite ingredients. In this chapter, we'll learn how to use hemp seed and oil, and how to incorporate our favorite CBD oil, CBD isolate, and water-soluble CBD into many recipes. Alcohol-free and totally sober treats that you and your guests will love!

Working with Culinary Hemp Seed and Hemp Seed Oil

As you have learned in the previous chapters, hemp seed and hemp seed oil are delicate culinary ingredients that require processing with low temperatures and have shorter shelf lives than many other oils and ingredients. In this chapter, you will pair edible recipes that have hemp seed and hemp seed oil with some of the whole aromatic spice and herb terpene blends you have explored in chapter 4 to create entourage effects for culinary and beverage creations.

Working with Off-the-Shelf CBD Products for Culinary Use

In this chapter, you will also incorporate your favorite CBD oils, extracts, and concentrates into edible recipes that also feature the whole aromatic spice and herb terpene blends from chapter 4. Off-the-shelf CBD oils, extracts, and concentrates have the advantage of being pre-decarboxylated (no need to heat in order to decarboxylate before use) and can be dosed exactly according to the milligrams of CBD printed on the ingredients label. For this reason, it's important to remember these products are also delicate ingredients that should not be exposed to heat for extended periods.

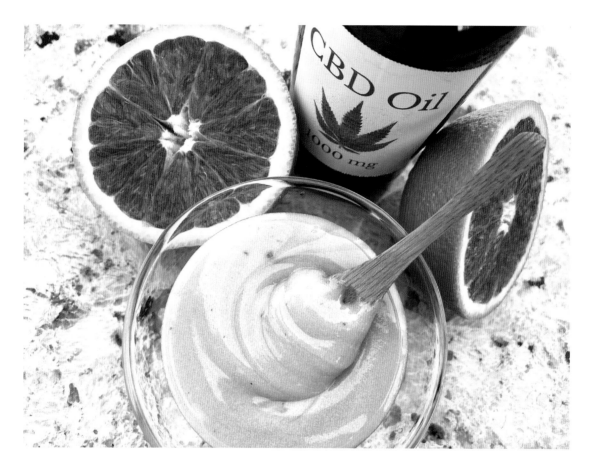

Honey Recipes

The benefits of honey come together with CBD and terpenes to create sweet, delicious, and therapeutic foods that are soothing and nourishing for both mind and body.

Herb, Fruit, and CBD–Infused Honey

A delightful honey recipe sure to become a kitchen staple! This honey can incorporate any terpene-rich herb, spice, or fruit blend. In this recipe, you may swap out the suggested herb, spice, and fruit blend and incorporate your favorite blend of terpene-rich ingredients. Enjoy this honey in tea, on your morning toast, or in any beverage or bakery item you would enjoy with plain honey.

Makes 16 ounces (480 ml) of infused honey

Instructions:

1. Boil/sterilize a quart (liter) canning jar and a pint (480 ml) canning jar. Allow both to dry.
2. In the quart canning jar, add all dry ingredients and then pour the honey over the top, covering them completely. Screw the top on the jar.
3. In a pan on the stove, add water and place the jar in the water. Bring the water to a boil and then immediately remove the pan from the stove. Allow the honey and spices to infuse until the water is cool. Remove the jar from water and allow it to dry.
4. Place the infusion jar in a dark cabinet to fully infuse all the terpenes from the spices into the honey for two weeks.
5. Bring out the jar of honey infusion and strain the honey from the spices into a sterilized pint canning jar.
6. Add the CBD oil to the infused honey and stir to combine thoroughly. A small whisk works well for this purpose. Affix the lid and use the honey within nine months for best results.

Ingredients:

Whole aromatic fruit, herb, spice blend (dried only), or your choice of dried whole aromatic spices from chapter 4 (page 47), such as: orange peels, lemon peels, star anise, white peppercorns, or cardamom pods, split

2 cups (480 ml) raw honey

1 ounce (30 ml) or less of your favorite CBD oil in the milligram dose you desire

Invigorating Lemon Mint Manuka Honey CBD–Infused Cough Drops

This cough drop brings together the benefits of both manuka honey and CBD to create a refreshing and soothing drop that you will surely want to stock up on for the winter season! Manuka honey is a special kind of honey produced from the single flowers of the Australian tea tree plant. This honey is usually sold in small amounts and is more expensive than other kinds of honey due to the amount produced in any given year and the unique properties of this honey.

Makes 30–60 cough drops depending on preferred size

Ingredients:

⅓ cup (80 ml) water
1 large handful of fresh mint leaves, chopped
Peels of 1 large lemon or 2 medium lemons, chopped
Juice from 1 large lemon or 2 medium lemons
1 cup (200 g) sugar
⅓ cup (80 ml) manuka honey
1 teaspoon (2 g) arrowroot powder dissolved in 1 teaspoon (5 ml) water
1–2 tablespoons (15–30 ml) or less of your favorite CBD oil, depending on the milligram serving size you desire for each cough drop

Instructions:

1. In a pan on the stove, add the water, mint leaves, and lemon peels. Turn on the heat and, as soon as the water starts to simmer, cover the pan, and turn off the heat. Allow the ingredients to infuse for an hour.

2. Strain the water from the plant material, making sure to squeeze out as much liquid as possible. Return the liquid to the pan on the stove and add the lemon juice and sugar. Stir to dissolve the sugar.

3. Cook on medium to medium-high until the temperature reaches 240° F (116° C) and then add the manuka honey. You will need a candy thermometer for this step and the next.

4. Continue cooking until the temperature reads 300° F (150° C) and then remove from the heat. Stir in the dissolved arrowroot powder and CBD oil immediately and distribute evenly throughout the mixture.

5. Working quickly using candy molds or a baking sheet lined with parchment paper, portion the mixture into individual servings. For best results, allow this to set for at least 6 hours before removing from molds or parchment paper. The cough drops can now be stored in an airtight container with a moisture-absorbing packet for extra moisture protection. Use within 3 months for best results.

Thief in the Night CBD–Infused Honey Pastilles

Based on the original recipe from the middle ages known as Vinegar of Four Thieves, this recipe uses lemon, cloves, and thyme as the herbal terpene blend to pair with your favorite CBD oil. Another favorite of the winter season and also great for traveling, these pastilles will freshen and soothe the mouth and throat when you need it most.

Makes 24–48 pastilles

Instructions:

1. In a pan on the stove, add the water, lemon juice, sugar, and honey. Stir to combine and then turn the heat to medium.
2. Cook on medium to medium-high, stirring constantly until the temperature reads 300° F (150° C) and then remove from the heat. You will need a candy thermometer for this step.
3. Stir in the essential oils and the CBD oil immediately and distribute evenly throughout the mixture.
4. Working quickly using candy molds or a baking sheet lined with parchment paper, portion the mixture into individual servings. For best results, allow this to set for at least 6 hours before removing from molds or parchment paper.
5. Place the pastilles in a bowl or bag with the powdered sugar and evenly coat all the surfaces. Store in a tightly sealed container, preferably with a moisture-absorbing pack. Use within 3 months for best results.

Ingredients:

¼ cup (60 ml) water
Juice from 1 large lemon or 2 medium lemons
½ cup (100 g) sugar
½ cup (120 ml) raw honey
1 drop clove essential oil
1 drop lavender essential oil
1 drop thyme essential oil
1 tablespoon (15 ml) or less of your favorite CBD oil, depending on the milligram serving size you desire for each pastille
Powdered sugar to coat the pastilles

Frankincense and Honey Pain–Relief Pastilles

Boswellia serrata, otherwise known as Indian frankincense, or just frankincense, is one of the many kinds of frankincense that are edible and used in many folk medicine recipes as an analgesic and anti-inflammatory. The compound in frankincense responsible for these effects is called boswellic acid. Boswellic acid only occurs in the whole resin of frankincense and never in the distilled essential oil because boswellic acid is a larger molecule unable to pass through the process of distillation used to make the essential oil. This recipe pairs whole frankincense resin with your favorite CBD oil to create a pain-relief pastille that really works!

Makes 24–48 pastilles depending on size

Ingredients:

¼ cup (60 ml) culinary orange flower water

Juice from 1 large lemon or 2 medium lemons

½ cup (100 g) sugar

½ cup (120 ml) raw honey

1 tablespoon (12 g) edible frankincense powder

1 tablespoon (15 ml) or less of your favorite CBD oil, depending on the milligram serving size you desire for each pastille

Powdered sugar to coat the pastilles

Instructions:

1. In a pan on the stove, add the orange flower water, lemon juice, sugar, honey, and frankincense powder. Stir to combine and then turn the heat to medium.
2. Cook on medium to medium-high, stirring constantly, until the temperature reads 300° F (150° C) and then remove from the heat. You will need a candy thermometer for this step.
3. Stir in the CBD oil immediately and distribute evenly throughout the mixture.
4. Working quickly using candy molds or a baking sheet lined with parchment paper, portion the mixture into individual servings. For best results, allow this to set for at least 6 hours before removing from molds or parchment paper.
5. Place the pastilles in a bowl or bag with the powdered sugar and evenly coat all of the surfaces. Store in a tightly sealed container, preferably with a moisture-absorbing pack. Use within 3 months for best results.

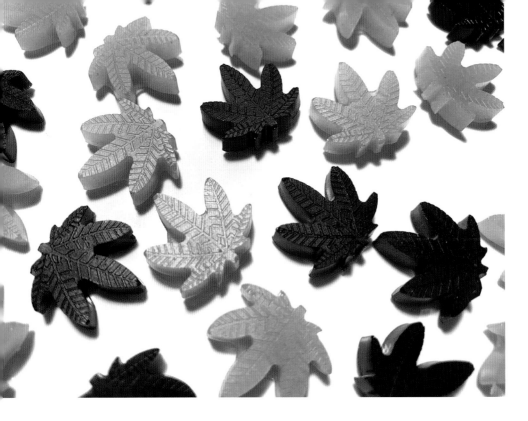

CBD Gummy Recipes

This CBD gummy guide will introduce you to two different ways to make gummies—and each will have their own unique texture based on the ingredients used. Try both methods and decide which textures you enjoy the most! Do you like a chewy, stretchy gummy? Then you may like gelatin gummies. Are vegan alternatives the best for you? You will prefer the agar-based gummies.

These gummy recipes all contain wholesome ingredients—but if you are on a sugar-restricted diet, you can also make these gummies with alternative sweeteners, such as stevia or erythritol.

No-Sugar CBD Gummies

A keto gummy that has zero carbs per serving. This gummy uses some fresh juice expressed from raspberries and lemons as the flavor base that will not affect blood-sugar levels. Rich in limonene terpene!

Makes 24–60 gummies depending on size.

Ingredients:

¼ cup (60 ml) lemon juice

Any sugar-free sweetener for the sweetness level you desire

2 tablespoons (20 g) unflavored gelatin, 250 bloom (preferably grass-fed beef)

¼ cup (60 ml) raspberry juice

Up to 2 teaspoons (10 ml) CBD oil (Calculate what the milligram serving size of CBD will be for each gummy.)

2 teaspoons (6 g) acacia fiber powder dissolved in 2 teaspoons (10 ml) of water

Instructions:

1. Divide the liquid into two parts. In the first part, combine the lemon juice and sugar-free sweetener. Stir until the sweetener is completely dissolved.

2. Add the gelatin to the raspberry juice, stir, and allow this to bloom. It will be thick and "rubbery" when bloomed. Set aside.

3. Pour the desired amount of CBD oil and the dissolved acacia fiber in a small cup and set aside.

4. In a small pan on the stove, add lemon juice mixture and warm it gently until it starts to steam.

5. Add the raspberry liquid with the bloomed gelatin to the hot lemon liquid on the stove and combine while cooking on medium-low until the gelatin completely dissolves into the hot liquid. Use a whisk or other vigorous stirring tool, if necessary. Do not allow it to boil.

6. Remove the hot gelatin liquid from the stove. Add the combined CBD oil and dissolved acacia fiber powder to the hot liquid and combine with the warm gelatin mixture using a whisk for best results.

7. Working quickly, use a kitchen syringe to pick up some of the liquid and fill the gummy molds. Do not wait to fill your molds, as the gummy

(Continued on page 138)

mixture will set up rather quickly. If the gummy mixture becomes too thick for the syringe, warm it again on the stove to liquify it.

8. Place the molded gummies in the freezer for 15 minutes, and then in the refrigerator for 1 hour to set them up.

9. Unmold all the gummies onto a piece of parchment or wax paper. Leave in the open air on the counter to allow them to dehydrate a bit for at least 3 hours.

10. The gummies are ready to go into a closed container at this point and should be refrigerated. Depending on the level of humidity in your environment, your gummies may benefit from a few more hours of drying in the open air. These gummies are best enjoyed within a month.

Spicy Golden Citrus Gummies

A delicious vegan gummy recipe that brings together the benefits of turmeric with CBD! Agar has a unique texture that is not "stretchy" like gelatin but is nonetheless still quite delicious. Try it and see what you think!

This recipe uses agar powder exclusively—other kinds of agar, such as flakes, will not form properly in this recipe.

Makes 24–60 gummies depending on size

Ingredients:

½ cup (120 ml) lemon juice

½ cup (100 g) sugar

1 teaspoon (3 g) turmeric powder

¼ tsp (0.5 g) black pepper

1½ tablespoons (15 g) agar powder

Up to 2 teaspoons (10 ml) CBD oil (Calculate what the milligram serving size of CBD will be for each gummy.)

Instructions:

1. In a pan on the stove, add the lemon juice, sugar, turmeric, and black pepper. Warm and stir until the sugar is dissolved.
2. Add the agar powder a little bit at a time while stirring. Lightly simmer for 5 minutes while stirring.
3. Remove from the heat and stir in the CBD oil. Allow to sit for 2 minutes and then stir again. Using a kitchen syringe, portion the liquid into the molds.
4. Place the tray of molds into the refrigerator and refrigerate for 2 hours. Unmold the gummies and store in a sealed container in the refrigerator for up to 2 weeks.

Clove-Pierced Blood Orange Gummies

Based on the Middle Ages remedy, in which a clove-pierced orange was carried in the pockets of monks, the clove-pierced orange remains today a favorite during the winter holidays for its spicy fragrance. This recipe turns this centuries-old fragrance pom into a delicious edible gummy recipe that tastes as good as it smells. Rich in terpenes—caryophyllene (clove) and myrcene (blood orange)—this gummy has an uplifting and potentiating entourage to accompany any dosage of CBD you select.

Makes approximately 20–50 depending on the size you prefer

Instructions:

1. In a bowl, combine the blood orange juice, clove, and sugar. Divide the liquid into two parts.
2. Add the gelatin to one part, stir and allow this to bloom. It will be thick and "rubbery" when bloomed.
3. In a small cup, pour the desired amount of CBD oil and the dissolved acacia fiber and set aside.
4. In a small pan on the stove, add the juice mixture (sans gelatin) and warm it gently until it starts to steam.
5. Add the juice with the bloomed gelatin to the hot juice liquid on the stove and combine while cooking on medium-low until the gelatin completely dissolves into the hot liquid. Use a whisk or other vigorous stirring tool, if necessary. Do not allow it to boil.
6. Remove the hot gelatin liquid from the stove. Add the combined CBD oil and dissolved acacia fiber powder and combine with the warm gelatin mixture using a whisk for best results.
7. Working quickly, use a kitchen syringe and fill the gummy molds. Do not wait to fill your molds, as the gummy mixture will set up rather

Ingredients:

½ cup (120 ml) blood orange juice*

¼ teaspoon (0.5 g) ground clove

1 tablespoon (10 g) sugar

2 tablespoons (20 g) unflavored gelatin, 250 bloom (preferably grass-fed beef)

Up to 2 teaspoons (10 ml) CBD oil (Calculate what the milligram serving size of CBD will be for each gummy.)

2 teaspoons (6 g) acacia fiber powder dissolved in 2 teaspoons (10 ml) water

Caster sugar to coat the outside, if desired

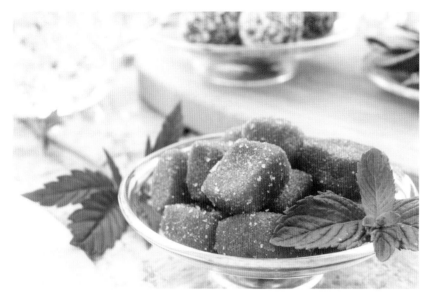

quickly. If the gummy mixture becomes too thick for the syringe, warm it again on the stove to liquify it.

8. Place the molded gummies in the freezer for 15 minutes, and then in the refrigerator for 1 hour to set them up.

9. Unmold all the gummies onto a piece of parchment or wax paper. Leave in the open air on the counter to allow them to dehydrate for at least 3 hours. After drying, sprinkle with caster sugar for extra sweetness and sparkle, if desired.

10. The gummies are ready to go into a closed container at this point and should be refrigerated. Depending on the level of humidity in your environment, your gummies may benefit from a few more hours of drying in the open air. These gummies are best enjoyed within a month.

---

* You may substitute regular orange juice for this recipe, but keep in mind that blood orange has more myrcene terpenes and makes a better CBD gummy.

Hot & Spicy Lime and Ginger Gummies

Another method to make gummies that works well with CBD oil is using a commercial gelatin dessert brand with sugar and citric acid already added to the mix along with grass-fed beef gelatin. To make this recipe, you can use any commercial brand that is plain with sugar and citric acid and citrus flavorings.

Makes 24–60 gummies depending on size

Instructions:

1. In a bowl, combine the ginger juice, lime juice, cayenne pepper, and sugar. Divide the liquid into two parts.
2. Add the unflavored gelatin to one part, stir, and allow this to bloom and set aside. It will be thick and "rubbery" when bloomed.
3. In a small cup, add the desired amount of CBD oil and the dissolved acacia fiber and set aside.
4. In a small pan on the stove, add the other half of the liquid and stir in the commercial powder gelatin dessert mix until it has dissolved and is hot.
5. Add the liquid with the bloomed gelatin to the hot liquid on the stove and stir until the gelatin completely dissolves into the hot liquid. Use a whisk or other vigorous stirring tool, if necessary. Do not allow it to boil.
6. Remove the hot gelatin liquid from the stove. Add the combined CBD oil and dissolved acacia fiber powder and bring together with the warm gelatin mixture using a whisk for best results.
7. Working quickly, use a kitchen syringe to fill the gummy molds. Do not wait to fill your molds, as the gummy mixture will set up quickly. If the gummy mixture becomes too thick for the syringe, warm it again on the stove to liquify it.

Ingredients:

2 tablespoons (30 ml) ginger juice

1 tablespoon (10 g) sugar or sugar-free sweetener equivalent

½ cup (120 ml) lime juice

¼ teaspoon (0.5 g) cayenne pepper (or more depending on how much heat you like)

1½ tablespoons (15 g) unflavored gelatin, 250 bloom (preferably grass-fed beef)

Up to 2 teaspoons (10 ml) CBD oil (Calculate what the milligram serving size of CBD will be for each gummy.)

2 teaspoons (6 g) acacia fiber powder dissolved in 2 teaspoons (10 ml) of water

1 tablespoons (10 g) plain commercial powder gelatin dessert mix

8. Place the molded gummies in the freezer for 15 minutes, and then in the refrigerator for 1 hour to set them up.
9. Unmold the gummies onto a piece of parchment or wax paper. Leave in the open air on the counter to allow them to dehydrate for at least 3 hours.
10. The gummies are ready to go into a closed container at this point and should be refrigerated. Depending on the level of humidity in your environment, your gummies may benefit from a few more hours of drying in the open air. These gummies are best enjoyed within a month.

Elderberry and Rose Gummies

This recipe uses the vegan formulation with agar powder. Elderberry is a favorite for cold and flu season and pairs with your favorite CBD oil for a supercharged home remedy everyone will appreciate! Remember to use agar powder only; flakes or other forms will not give the same results.

Makes 24–60 gummies depending on size

Instructions:

1. In a pan on the stove, add the elderberry juice and the sugar. Warm and stir until the sugar is dissolved.
2. Add the agar powder a little bit at a time while stirring. Lightly simmer for 5 minutes while stirring.
3. Remove from the heat and stir in the rose water and the CBD oil. Allow to sit for 2 minutes and then stir again. Using a kitchen syringe, portion the liquid into the molds.
4. Place the tray of molds into the refrigerator and refrigerate for 2 hours. Unmold the gummies and store in a sealed container in the refrigerator for up to 2 weeks.

Ingredients:

½ cup (120 ml) elderberry juice
3 tablespoons (30 g) sugar
1½ tablespoons (15 g) agar powder
1 tablespoon (15 ml) culinary rose water
Up to 2 teaspoons (10 ml) CBD oil (Calculate what the milligram serving size of CBD will be for each gummy.)

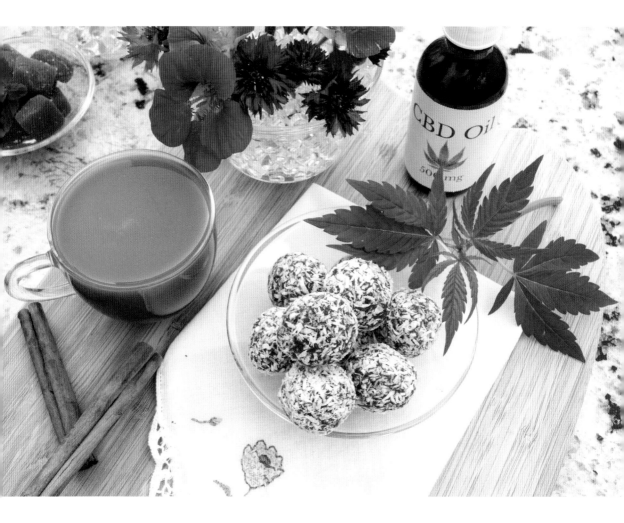

Hemp and CBD No-Bake Bite Recipes

Here are three recipes for delicious little healthy and happy treats that bring together all the benefits of CBD and hemp seed! These bites can be served any time of day. You may also omit the CBD oil and just make these with hemp seed, if you desire.

Coconut Hemp Brownie Bites

Probably the easiest and most delicious brownie recipe in the world! These aren't the brownies you remember from your college dorm—and they won't get you high. You can still enjoy all the benefits of cannabis with these CBD-infused brownies that you can make in 15 minutes and don't require baking.

Makes about 12–24 brownie bites depending on size

Instructions:

1. In a bowl, combine the softened coconut butter with the CBD oil.
2. In a food processor, add the pitted dates, coconut butter/CBD oil, vanilla extract, and the powdered cocoa, and begin to process until almost a dough. Add the shelled hemp seed and continue processing until everything is thoroughly combined. Add half the coconut flakes and process until combined.
3. On a board or baking sheet lined with parchment paper, roll out the dough and coat with the rest of the coconut flakes. Cut into little bites.
4. Refrigerate for 1 hour until firm. Transfer to a sealed container. These can be stored in a sealed container for up to 3 weeks in the refrigerator.

Ingredients:

⅓ cup (150 g) softened coconut butter

1 tablespoon (15 ml) or less of your favorite CBD oil, depending on the milligram serving size you desire for each brownie

2 cups (350 g) soft pitted dates

1 teaspoon (5 ml) vanilla extract

¼ cup (25 g) powdered cocoa

1 cup (240 g) shelled hemp seed

½ cup (35 g) coconut flakes, divided

Oatmeal Cookie Bites

Everyone loves oatmeal cookies, and these sweet treats will be ready in a snap! This recipe uses the Harvest Spice terpene blend from chapter 4 as an entourage for your hemp and CBD experience.

Makes about 12–24 oatmeal cookie bites depending on size

Ingredients:

⅔ cup (150 g) almond butter

1 tablespoon (15 ml) or less of your favorite CBD oil, depending on the milligram serving size you desire for each cookie bite

⅔ cup (135 g) dark brown sugar

½ teaspoon (1 g) salt

1 teaspoon (5 ml) vanilla extract

1 teaspoon (3 g) Harvest Spice (page 48)

⅓ cup (80 g) shelled hemp seed

¾ cup (65 g) rolled oats

Instructions:

1. In a bowl, combine the almond butter with the CBD oil.
2. In another bowl, combine the brown sugar, salt, vanilla extract, and the Harvest Spice blend. Add the almond butter mixture to this and bring together using a hand mixer or stand mixer.
3. Add the hemp seed and the rolled oats and thoroughly combine with the almond butter and sugar mixture.
4. On a board or baking sheet lined with parchment paper, roll out the dough and cut into little bites.
5. Refrigerate for 1 hour until firm. Transfer to a sealed container. These can be stored in a sealed container for up to 2 weeks in the refrigerator.

Holiday Fruitcake Bites

What if you could make a fruitcake recipe for the holiday season that everyone would love? Fruitcake will have a great reputation this holiday season, because instead of making it with that weird candied fruit with artificial flavoring, these fruitcake bites feature real dried fruit and a terpene entourage to pair with CBD and hemp.

Makes about 12–24 fruitcake bites

Instructions:

1. In a bowl, combine the coconut butter with the CBD oil.
2. In another bowl, combine the brown sugar, salt, vanilla extract, and the Gingerbread House spice blend. Add the coconut butter mixture to this and bring together using a hand mixer or stand mixer.
3. Add the hemp seed, almond flour, and dried fruits and thoroughly combine with the coconut butter/sugar mixture.
4. On a board or baking sheet lined with parchment paper, roll out the dough, cut into little bites, and dust with powdered sugar.
5. Refrigerate for 1 hour until firm. Transfer to a sealed container. These can be stored in a sealed container for up to 3 weeks in the refrigerator.

Ingredients:

½ cup (150 g) coconut butter

1 tablespoon (15 ml) or less of your favorite CBD oil, depending on the milligram serving size you desire for each fruitcake bite

¾ cup (150 g) light brown sugar

½ teaspoon (1 g) salt

1 teaspoon (5 ml) vanilla extract

2 teaspoons (6 g) Gingerbread House spice blend (page 53)

⅓ cup (80 g) shelled hemp seed

¾ cup (80 g) almond flour

⅔ cup (50 g) assorted dried fruits such as golden berries, apricots, goji berries, cherries, etc.

Powdered sugar for dusting

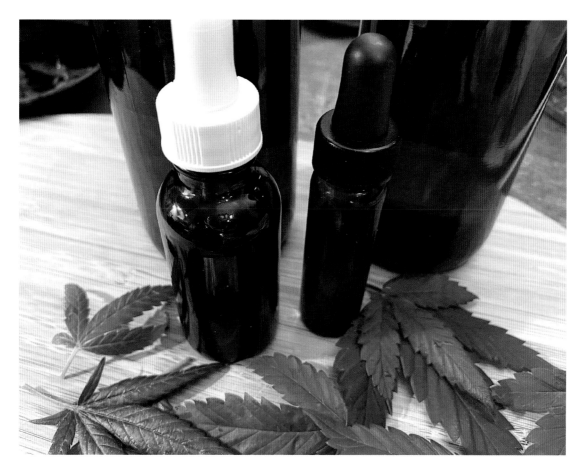

CBD Tinctures and Bitters

Tincturing is a traditional herbal medicinal art form that goes back at least one thousand years to the age of alchemy. These tinctures are basic tinctures that you can make easily with herbs, high-proof alcohol, and your favorite CBD extract or oil. The recipes here are basic enough that you can swap out ingredients and try new blends that you enjoy. Like the other recipes, these tinctures are formulated based on herbal terpene entourage paired with CBD.

Digestive Bitters

The most well-known type of tincture in the world is the digestive bitter. This tincture is commonly taken after meals, especially heavy meals, to soothe the stomach and aid digestion.

Makes 1 (4-ounce/120 ml) tincture

Instructions:

1. Boil/sterilize an amber glass dropper bottle and glass dropper, and allow to dry. Affix the dropper to the lid and set aside until the tincture is ready in 3 weeks.
2. In a clean glass canning jar, add all ingredients except for the CBD oil or extract. Affix the lid, shake the jar, and put in a cool, dark cabinet for 3 weeks.
3. Decant the tincture and strain the herbs from the alcohol. Pour the tincture into the amber glass bottle and add the CBD oil or extract. Affix the dropper lid and shake the bottle. Use within 6 months for best results.

How to use:

Shake the bottle before each use, draw up the amount of tincture into the dropper, and consume directly or add to hot liquids such as hot lemon water.

Ingredients:

½ cup 100-proof alcohol
Peels from 1 large orange or 2 medium oranges, chopped
1 tablespoon (3 g) fennel seeds
1 tablespoon (3 g) angelica seed
1 teaspoon (2 g) fenugreek seed
1 teaspoon (2 g) powdered ginger root
2 teaspoons (10 ml) or less of your favorite CBD oil, depending on the milligram serving size you desire for each dropper-sized serving of tincture

Relaxation Tincture

Relieve stress and rest easy with this unique tincture, which pairs relaxing terpenes and other herbal compounds with CBD. It's a relaxation tincture that will relieve stress when you need to stay awake but can also be used as a sleep aid for nap time or nighttime.

Makes 1 (4 ounce/120 ml) tincture

Ingredients:

½ cup 100-proof alcohol

2 tablespoons (5 g) dried lemon balm (melissa) herb

2 tablespoons (5 g) dried lavender flowers

1 tablespoon (3 g) dried chamomile flowers

1 tablespoon (3 g) dried hibiscus flowers

2 teaspoons (10 ml) or less of your favorite CBD oil, depending on the milligram serving size you desire for each dropper-sized serving of tincture

Instructions:

1. Boil/sterilize an amber glass dropper bottle and glass dropper, and allow to dry. Affix the dropper to the lid and set aside until the tincture is ready in 3 weeks.
2. In a clean glass canning jar, add all the ingredients except for the CBD oil or extract. Affix the lid, shake the jar, and put in a cool, dark cabinet for 3 weeks.
3. Decant the tincture and strain the herbs from the alcohol. Pour the tincture into the amber glass bottle and add the CBD oil or extract. Affix the dropper lid and shake the bottle. Use within 6 months for best results.

How to use:

Shake the bottle before each use, draw up the amount of tincture into the dropper, and consume directly or add to hot liquids such as hot lemon water.

Energizing Tincture

Refresh and revitalize with this tincture in your morning tea! This tincture is caffeine-free and can be used in any hot beverage whenever you need an energizing pick-me-up.

Makes 1 (4 ounces/120 ml) tincture

Instructions:

1. Boil/sterilize an amber glass dropper bottle and glass dropper, and allow to dry. Affix the dropper to the lid and set aside until the tincture is ready in 3 weeks.
2. In a clean glass canning jar, add the ingredients except for the CBD oil or extract. Affix the lid, shake the jar, and put in a cool, dark cabinet for 3 weeks.
3. Decant the tincture and strain the herbs from the alcohol. Pour the tincture into the amber glass bottle and add the CBD oil or extract. Affix the dropper lid and shake the bottle. Use within 6 months for best results.

How to use:

Shake the bottle before each use, draw up the amount of tincture into the dropper, and consume directly or add to hot liquids such as hot lemon water.

Ingredients:

½ cup 100-proof alcohol

Peels from 1 large lemon or 2 medium lemons, chopped

1 tablespoon (3 g) ashwagandha root powder

1 tablespoon (3 g) maca root powder

1 small ginseng root (about the size of your thumb or smaller), chopped

2 teaspoons (4 g) powdered ginger root

2 teaspoons (10 ml) or less of your favorite CBD oil, depending on the milligram serving size you desire for each dropper-sized serving of tincture

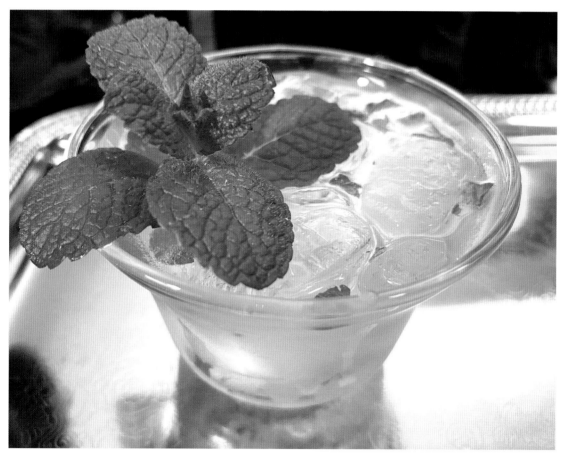

CBD Mocktails and Beverages

Simple yet elegant beverages you can enjoy every day or prepare for your guests. These beverages are prepared with your favorite water-soluble CBD extract and paired with fruit, flowers, and herbs rich in aromatic plant terpenes.

Fresh Mint and Lime Mojito

An alcohol-free "mocktail" that's sober, fun, and relaxing, too. Perfect for a girls' night in or any festive gathering.

Makes about 4 "mocktails," depending on the serving size of your cocktail glasses

Instructions:

1. Juice all the limes in a glass measuring cup or other container. Cut 4 small slices of lime for garnish.
2. In each cocktail glass, add even amounts of the lime juice, sugar or sweetener, and the water-soluble CBD extract. Combine all of this thoroughly in the bottom of each glass.
3. Add the desired amount of mint leaves per glass and lightly crush and bruise them into the liquid in the bottom of the glass.
4. Add the crushed ice to each glass, add the carbonated mineral water, and stir to combine everything. Garnish with a lime slice and serve immediately.

Ingredients:

4 large limes, juiced
Sugar or sugar-free sweetener, to taste
The desired amount of your favorite water-soluble CBD extract per glass
1 handful fresh mint leaves
Crushed ice
Carbonated mineral water

Rose Lemonade

A delightful and cooling lemonade that will quench whole-body thirst. Prepared as a sugar-free beverage, it's an excellent thirst-quencher after hiking or working out. It's also an impressive beverage to serve guests that can be prepared quickly!

Makes about 1 quart (1 liter)

Ingredients:

2 large or 4 medium whole lemons, juiced

2 tablespoons (30 ml) culinary rose water

1 teaspoon (5 ml) beet juice or other natural pink food coloring (for a pretty pink color)

Sugar or sugar-free sweetener for the sweetness level you desire

1 teaspoon (5 ml) or less of your favorite water-soluble CBD extract

1 quart (1 liter) cold sparkling mineral water

Fresh roses or rose petals from the garden to float on the lemonade in a pitcher

Instructions:

1. Juice the lemons. Add the lemon juice, rose water, beet juice or other natural coloring, the sweetener of your choice, and the CBD extract to your beverage-serving pitcher. Whisk vigorously to combine.
2. Add the sparkling mineral water and stir. Fill with ice if you prefer.
3. Float the fresh roses or rose petals on top and serve immediately.

Elderflower Cordial

Elderflower cordial is a traditional European beverage syrup that can be enjoyed in plain or sparkling water—it's also delicious in cold or hot green tea! This recipe will make the syrup, and then you can add it to the beverage or water of your choice.

Makes about 6 ounces (150 ml)

Instructions:

1. In a pan on the stove, add the water, elderflowers, and lemon peels and juice. Simmer for 15 to 20 minutes until the water level drops about 10%. Turn off the heat and allow the liquid to cool completely.
2. Strain the liquid from the plant material and return the liquid to the pan. Add the sugar and stir. Turn on the heat and reduce the liquid to about half, at which point it will be a syrup. Remove from the heat.
3. Allow the cordial syrup to cool, and then add the CBD extract and combine thoroughly. Pour the syrup into a canning jar or bottle, and store in the refrigerator for up to 2 months.

How to use:

Spoon the syrup into sparkling water, plain water, or tea, and enjoy.

Ingredients:

1½ cups (360 ml) water
½ cup (40 g) dried elderflowers
1 large or 2 medium lemon peels and juice
¾ cup (150 g) sugar
2 teaspoons (10 ml) or less of your favorite water-soluble CBD extract

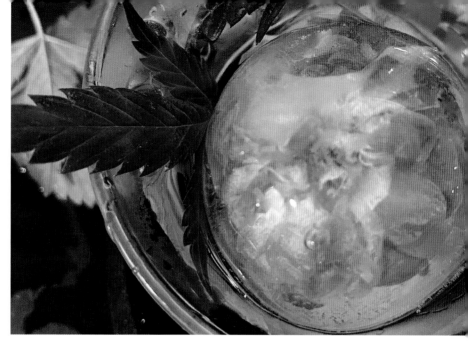

CBD & Terpenes Ice Cubes and Sculptures

CBD pairs with fruit, flower, and herbal terpenes in totally easy recipes that look as stunning as they taste! These recipes use either your favorite water-soluble CBD extracts or CBD-infused bottled water. Both of these products can be found at many retail stores that carry CBD oils, extracts, and other products.

To make this ice, you can use regular cube trays or you can use ice molds in various shapes, such as sculptures or spheres. These ice cubes and sculptures are a gracious idea for serving water or drinks of any kind at your next gathering. The techniques for each recipe feature a decorative placement of fruit and herbs in the ice cubes and sculptures for impressive service. These recipes use distilled water and a slow-freezing technique to create the clearest ice possible. Keep in mind that because you are using a CBD extract in the water, the ice may not be totally clear, but it will have more clarity than if you used plain tap or spring water.

Floral & Citrus Ice

Makes as many cubes or sculptures as you desire

Instructions:

1. Prechill your ice cube or sculpture molds in the freezer. Don't take them out until you're ready to fill them.
2. Boil a pan of distilled water twice for 5 minutes each boil. Allow the water to cool between each boiling.
3. After the water has cooled from the second boil to a warm temperature, stir in the amount of CBD extract or CBD-infused bottled water that you desire based on the milligram serving you want for each cube or sculpture. Allow this to sit on the counter for 30 minutes and then put in the refrigerator for 1 hour to chill.
4. Prepare the sculpture molds by placing flower and citrus arrangements in each one. Take the cold water out of the refrigerator and give it a quick, gentle stir. Using a spoon or small measuring cup, pour the cold water into each mold and then gently tap it on the counter to release air bubbles that may form during the process.
5. Your freezer should be set to the lowest temperature and freezing the cubes or sculptures should take about a day—this slow-freeze process will help create a clear ice. Place the molds in the freezer and allow to freeze solid. Serve as desired.

Ingredients:

Distilled water
Water-soluble CBD extract or CBD-infused bottled water
Fresh edible flowers and citrus (petals such as rose petals, citrus flowers, carnation petals, etc. and any citrus cut into very thin decorative slices)

Green Tea & Mint Ice

Makes as many cubes or sculptures as you desire

Ingredients:

Distilled water
Green tea bags
Water-soluble CBD
    extract or CBD-
    infused bottled water
Fresh mint leaves (not
    wilted)

Instructions:

1. Prechill your ice cube or sculpture molds in the freezer. Don't take them out until you're ready to fill them.

2. Boil a pan of distilled water for 5 minutes. Boil a second time for 5 minutes, and remove from the heat.

3. Rinse one or more green tea bags in cool water and then add them to the hot water that you just boiled and removed from the heat. Allow these to steep for 2 minutes and then remove the tea bags and allow the water to cool to a warm temperature.

4. After the water has cooled to a warm temperature, stir in the amount of CBD extract or CBD-infused bottled water that you desire based on the milligram serving you want for each cube or sculpture. Allow this to sit on the counter for 30 minutes and then put in the refrigerator for 1 hour to chill.

5. Prepare the sculpture molds by placing mint leaf arrangements in each one. Take the cold tea-infused water out of the refrigerator and give it a quick, gentle stir. Using a spoon or small measuring cup, pour the cold liquid into each mold and then gently tap it on the counter to release air bubbles that may form during the process.

6. Your freezer should be set to the lowest temperature and freezing the cubes or sculptures should take about a day—this slow-freeze process will help create a clear ice. Place the molds in the freezer and allow to freeze solid. Serve as desired.

Ginger Mango Ice

Makes as many cubes or sculptures as you desire

Instructions:

1. Prechill your ice cube or sculpture molds in the freezer. Don't take them out until you're ready to fill them.
2. Boil a pan of distilled water twice for 5 minutes each boil. Allow the water to cool between each boiling.
3. After the water has cooled from the second boil to a warm temperature, stir in the amount of CBD extract or CBD-infused bottled water that you desire based on the milligram serving you want for each cube or sculpture. Allow this to sit on the counter for 30 minutes and then put in the refrigerator for 1 hour to chill.
4. Prepare the sculpture molds by placing ginger and mango arrangements in each one. Take the cold water out of the refrigerator and give it a quick, gentle stir. Using a spoon or small measuring cup, pour the cold water into each mold and then gently tap it on the counter to release air bubbles that may form during the process.
5. Your freezer should be set to the lowest temperature, and freezing the cubes or sculptures should take about a day—this slow-freeze process will help create a clear ice. Place the molds in the freezer and allow to freeze solid. Serve as desired.

Ingredients:

Distilled water
Water-soluble CBD extract or CBD-infused bottled water
Fresh slices of ginger and firm mango cut thinly or in decorative shapes

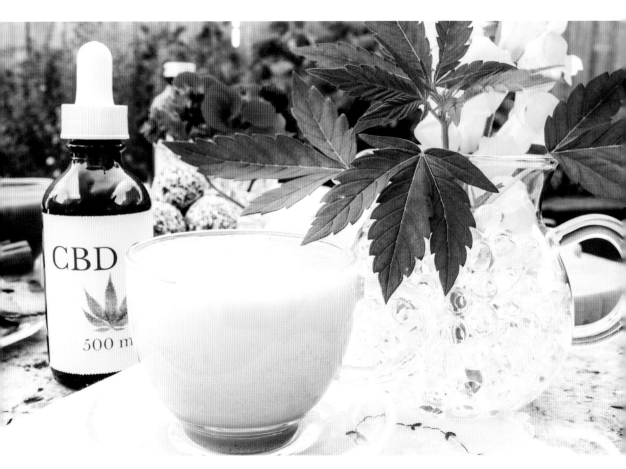

Pictured above, Classic Golden Milk

Nourishing Hemp and CBD Smoothies and Drinks

These are nutritious hot drinks and creamy smoothies featuring hemp seed and your favorite CBD oil. These CBD recipes can be made in less than 5 minutes and feature entourage ingredients to enhance your CBD experience.

Classic Golden Milk

A classic Ayurvedic favorite that tastes great. This hot drink features a soothing spice blend entourage that pairs perfectly with your favorite CBD oil.

Makes about 8 ounces (240 ml)

Instructions:

1. In a pan on the stove, gently warm the milk, Golden Blend, and sweetener on medium heat until hot. Remove from the stove immediately.
2. Pour into a cup and stir in the desired amount of CBD oil. Serve immediately.

Ingredients:

1 cup (240 ml) whole dairy milk or vegan extra-cream coconut milk

1 teaspoon (3 g) Golden Blend (page 51)

Sugar or sugar-free sweetener to taste

1 teaspoon (5 ml) or less of your favorite CBD oil

Rose and Cardamom Milk

A beautiful beverage that is floral, fragrant, and spicy with terpenes of caryophyllene and myrcene from the cardamom pod, a spice in the ginger family.

Makes about 8 ounces (240 ml)

Instructions:

1. In a pan on the stove gently warm the milk, crushed cardamom, sweetener, and pinch of beet powder on medium heat until hot. Remove from the stove immediately.
2. Pour into a cup and stir in the rose water and desired amount of CBD oil. Serve immediately.

Ingredients:

1 cup (240 ml) whole dairy milk or vegan extra cream coconut milk

2 cardamom pods, seeds removed and crushed

Sugar or sugar-free sweetener to taste

Pinch beet powder for pink color

1 tablespoon (15 ml) culinary rose water

1 teaspoon (5 ml) or less of your favorite CBD oil

Ingredients:

2 medium bananas
1 teaspoon (3 g) Golden Blend (page 51)
1 teaspoon (5 ml) vanilla extract
3–6 seedless dates based on the sweetness level you desire
⅓ cup (80 g) shelled hemp seed
1 cup (200 g) ice chips
1 teaspoon (5 ml) or less of your favorite CBD oil

Golden Banana Smoothie

A cool, vegan smoothie based on the traditional golden milk recipe featuring the benefits of turmeric, CBD, and the superfood nutrition of dates and hemp seed. This smoothie is a great way to energize and start the day!

Makes about 12 ounces (360 ml)

Instructions:

Everything goes into the blender and blend until creamy. Enjoy!

Ingredients:

½ cup (120 ml) sour cherry juice
1 tablespoon (15 ml) lime juice
Sugar or sugar-free sweetener to taste
⅓ cup (80 g) shelled hemp seed
1 cup (200 g) ice chips
1 teaspoon (5 ml) or less of your favorite CBD oil

Tart Cherry Limeade Smoothie

Sour cherries are often considered a superfood due to their benefits for inflammation. This recipe brings together sour cherry with both hemp seed and CBD for a super-nutritious smoothie that tastes as good as it is good for you.

Makes about 12 ounces (360 ml)

Instructions:

Everything goes into the blender and blend until creamy. Enjoy!

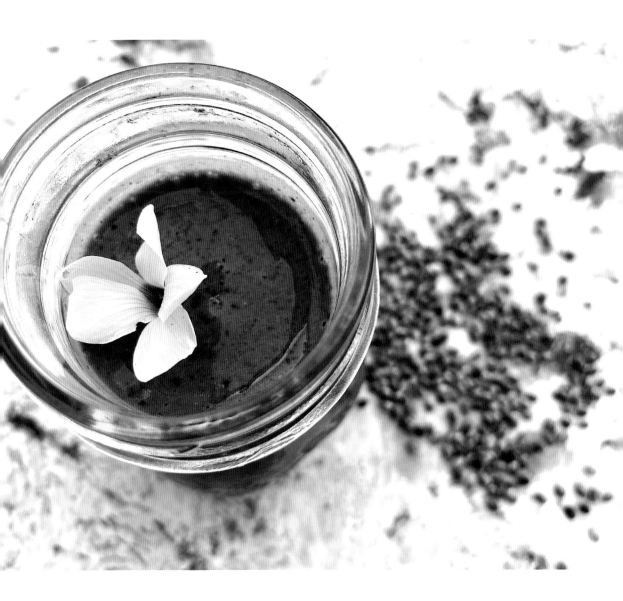

Ingredients:

⅔ cup (130 g) ice chips
2 tablespoons (30 ml)
  water
1 cup (150 g) blackberries
1 teaspoon (5 ml) vanilla
  extract
⅓ cup (80 g) shelled
  hemp seed
Sugar-free sweetener to
  taste
1 teaspoon (5 ml) or less
  of your favorite CBD
  oil

Vanilla Blackberry Keto Smoothie

Blackberries are a low-carb fruit favored by many people who follow low-carb and keto diets. This smoothie has the yummy flavor of a blackberry muffin but without the carbs!

Makes about 12 ounces (360 ml)

Instructions:

Everything goes into the blender and blend until creamy. Enjoy!

RESOURCE GUIDE

Most recipes in this book use ingredients found at your regular grocer, big-box retailer, or natural grocers. For some specialty ingredients, check out some of my personal sourcing recommendations:

Amazon.com
Amazon carries every specialty and organic ingredient you can't find locally.

Persian Basket—persianbasket.com
A personal favorite of mine, especially for spices, dates, and culinary floral water of every kind.

CBD Products, Oils, Etc.
I am neutral on this—see the first two chapters for advice on selecting and testing these products and choosing your preferred brands.

Cannabis Flower Essence—cannabisfloweressence.com
If you're interested in purchasing a commercial brand instead of making your own.

Reliable CBD information—projectcbd.com
One of the better sources of information about CBD. This is a noncommercial website.

Author's website, posy & kettle —posyandkettle.com
Visit this website and find out more about the author's books and the things she makes.

ABOUT THE AUTHOR

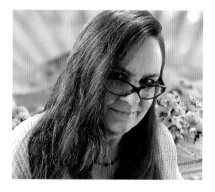

SANDRA HINCHLIFFE is the founder of posyandkettle.com, artisan herbalist, allergy chef, autoimmune disease survivor, and an inventor of pretty things for people of sensitive constitution. She uses her background as a herbalist and medical cannabis patient to create a repertoire of recipes designed to be both beneficial and delightful. She is the author of *CBD and Hemp Remedies*, a guide and recipe book for hemp and hemp product consumers; *CBD Every Day*, a celebration of farm-to-table CBD-rich cannabis; *The Cannabis Spa at Home*, the first book to bring together cannabis, spa, and herbal healing; and *High Tea*, a collection of wellness recipes for every occasion. She resides in Del Norte County, California.

CONVERSION CHARTS

Metric and Imperial Conversions

(These conversions are rounded for convenience)

Ingredient	Cups/ Tablespoons/ Teaspoons	Ounces	Grams/ Milliliters
Fruit, dried	1 cup	4 ounces	120 grams
Fruits or veggies, chopped	1 cup	5 to 7 ounces	145 to 200 grams
Fruits or veggies, puréed	1 cup	8.5 ounces	245 grams
Honey, maple syrup, or corn syrup	1 tablespoon	0.75 ounce	20 grams (15 milliliters)
Liquids: cream, milk, water, or juice	1 cup	8 fluid ounces	240 milliliters
Salt	1 teaspoon	0.2 ounces	6 grams
Spices: cinnamon, cloves, ginger, or nutmeg (ground)	1 teaspoon	0.2 ounce	5 milliliters (2 grams)
Sugar, brown, firmly packed	1 cup	7 ounces	200 grams
Sugar, white	1 cup/ 1 tablespoon	7 ounces/0.5 ounce	200 grams/12.5 grams
Vanilla extract	1 teaspoon	0.2 ounce	4 grams (5 milliliters)

Liquids

8 fluid ounces = 1 cup = ½ pint

16 fluid ounces = 2 cups = 1 pint

32 fluid ounces = 4 cups = 1 quart

128 fluid ounces = 16 cups = 1 gallon

INDEX